AIDS BIBLIOGRAPHY SERIES

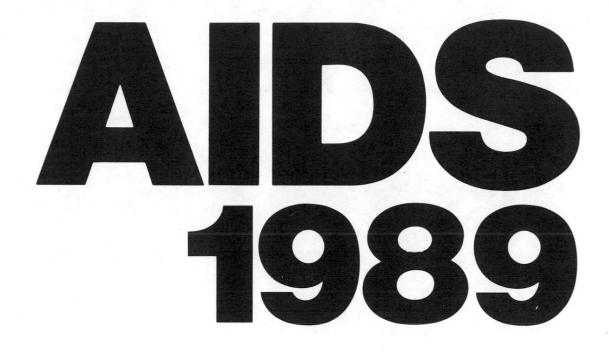

AIDS 1989

Part 1

by David A. Tyckoson

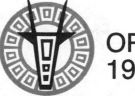
ORYX PRESS
1990

The rare Arabian Oryx is believed to have inspired the myth of the unicorn. This desert antelope became virtually extinct in the early 1960s. At that time several groups of international conservationists arranged to have 9 animals sent to the Phoenix Zoo to be the nucleus of a captive breeding herd. Today the Oryx population is nearly 800, and over 400 have been returned to reserves in the Middle East.

Copyright © 1990 by David A. Tyckoson
Published by The Oryx Press
2214 North Central at Encanto
Phoenix, Arizona 85004-1483

Published simultancously in Canada

Printed and Bound in the United States of America

The paper used in this publication meets the minimum requirements of American National Standard for Information Science—Permanence of Paper for Printed Library Materials, ANSI Z39.48, 1984.

ISBN 0-89774-578-7
ISSN 0899-9449

Table of Contents

Oryx AIDS Bibliographies
by David A. Tyckoson

AIDS 1986
AIDS 1987
AIDS 1988, Part 1
AIDS 1988, Part 2
AIDS 1989, Part 1

Forthcoming:

AIDS 1989, Part 2

Also Forthcoming from The Oryx Press:

The AIDS Information Sourcebook, Third Edition
by H. Robert Malinowsky and Gerald J. Perry

About the Series

The <u>AIDS Bibliography</u> series published by Oryx Press is designed to collect and evaluate the most significant material covering all aspects of the AIDS crisis. Issued semi-annually, each bibliography will contain references to approximately 500 of the most significant articles on the scientific, social, and ethical aspects of AIDS. A "Research Review" is also included to summarize progress in AIDS research during the time period covered by the bibliography. Taken individually, these bibliographies provide the user with an introduction to the research and issues surrounding the AIDS epidemic during the time period covered. Taken collectively, they represent a chronicle of the history of AIDS and demonstrate the changes in the trends and issues associated with the disease. Each bibliography also contains a number of special features, including:

Evaluative Selection. The bibliographer reviews each article to ensure that only the most valuable references are included. The bibliography does not strive to be comprehensive, but to include only the most important or most representative items on each topic.

Fully Annotated. All references selected for inclusion are annotated, providing the reader with a summary of the source material.

Readily Available Sources. All references selected for inclusion in the bibliography are available at most libraries throughout the United States and Canada. Obscure sources that are difficult to obtain are generally avoided.

Key Articles Highlighted. The most significant sources in each bibliography (as chosen by the compiler) are highlighted in **boldface** so that the user interested in only a few articles can key into those that are the most useful.

Undergraduate Reading Level. Only materials written at the undergraduate student level are selected. Articles that are highly technical or extremely general are usually avoided.

English Language Only. Only articles written in the English language are included in each bibliography.

Research Review. Each issue contains a research review summarizing the progress in the fight against AIDS and highlighting the key issues related to the disease.

Research Review: AIDS Update

The mood surrounding the AIDS crisis remained grim during the second half of 1988. While AIDS research continued at a steady pace, no significant breakthroughs were reported. The number of cases continues to rise at a dramatic rate and no cure or treatment has yet been discovered. Research on vaccines against the AIDS virus is progressing very slowly, although some human trials are currently in progress. While there is optimism that AIDS will be defeated at some time in the future, that time does not appear imminent.

Epidemiology of AIDS

The worldwide number of AIDS cases doubles every year. Over 100,000 cases have been reported worldwide and at least ten million other persons have been infected by the AIDS virus. Research indicates that all persons who become infected will contract the disease and that all persons who contract the disease will die of AIDS. Unless a cure or vaccine is discovered soon, the numbers of AIDS deaths will rise rapidly over the next few years.

On a geographic basis, the United States still contains the vast majority of all AIDS cases reported worldwide. North America accounts for 74% of all AIDS cases, with the United States alone representing almost 70% of all cases. European nations have reported 13% of the world's total number of cases, with another 12% reported in Africa. Asia and Oceania remain the least affected by AIDS, accounting for less than 1% of the world's total. However, these statistics may be skewed by the under-reporting of AIDS cases in several Third World nations. Scientists believe that several African and Caribbean nations are denying the existence of AIDS in their countries for political reasons. For example, no new AIDS cases have been reported in Zaire since the 335 known as of June 1987. Projections based on computer models of the epidemic indicate that at least 50,000 new cases probably have occurred in this nation alone during the last two years. Because of under-reporting, the reality of the AIDS crisis may be even worse than the current statistics indicate.

In the United States and Europe, the disease remains concentrated within several high risk groups. In the United States, homosexual men account for 63% of all AIDS cases, intravenous drug users represent 20% of the cases, and homosexual men who are also intravenous drug users account for 7% of AIDS cases. Sexual partners of AIDS victims represent 5% and blood transfusion recipients and hemophiliacs 2% of all American AIDS cases. No risk factors have been identified in a total of 339 AIDS victims, but researchers believe that further investigation would reveal that most infected persons fall into one of the above categories. Over 9% of all AIDS victims are women and slightly less than 2% of AIDS victims are children.

The AIDS epidemic in Africa and other Third World nations demonstrates a distinctly different epidemiological pattern than that shown in the United States. AIDS affects men and women in nearly equal numbers in Africa. Research strongly indicates that heterosexual transmission is the primary pathway for the virus in African nations. African AIDS cases are found primarily in urban areas and along major transportation routes, leaving rural areas virtually unaffected. In addition to heterosexual transmission, contaminated blood and blood products contribute to the transmission of the virus in the Third World. Both of these pathways will be difficult to eliminate in developing nations due to the expense of AIDS blood testing, the generally less developed health care facilities and systems, and the cultural factors surrounding human sexuality.

The Medical and Health Care Aspects of AIDS

The clinical definition of the disease remains virtually unchanged. Researchers have been able to precisely define the disease throughout all of its stages. Initial infection by the AIDS virus produces no symptoms in the victim. The virus remains latent within the body for several years. During this time period it reproduces and attacks the helper T-cells that comprise the body's immune system. As the immune system becomes weakened, the body becomes subject to a series of secondary infections from any of several other agents, including pneumocystis carinii pneumonia, Kaposi's sarcoma, tuberculosis, cytomegalovirus, and mycobacterium avium intracellulare. While the body may recover from any one of these infections, it is continually weakened and becomes more susceptible to future infections. This series of secondary infections eventually leads to the death of the patient. AIDS patients do not die directly from infection by the AIDS virus, but from this constant progression of other infections.

In addition to weakening the immune system and leaving the body open to secondary infections, the virus also directly infects the nervous system. The virus attack the brain directly and can cause AIDS dementia, in which the victim's mental functions are slowly destroyed over time. Many AIDS victims fear the neurological implications of infection with the AIDS virus more than they fear the secondary infections from other agents.

Some researchers have tried to link infection by the AIDS virus with syphilis. Since both diseases attack the brain as well as the body, researchers theorize that there may be a common method of fighting both conditions. In addition, men who have had syphilis at any time during their lives are much more likely to develop AIDS, even when they have been completely cured of syphilis. It is not clear how the two diseases interact (if at all), but researchers are studying the relationship between AIDS and syphilis in hopes of finding a clue to stopping the spread of each disease.

Zidovudine as a Therapy for AIDS

To date, only one drug therapy has been proven effective for use with AIDS patients. Zidovudine, formerly known as azidothymidine or AZT, has been shown to stop the progression of the disease among AIDS patients suffering from pneumocystis carinii pneumonia. The initial study on the effectiveness of zidovudine was so successful that it was halted in midstream in order to make the drug available to all members of the study group. Although zidovudine stops the reproduction of the AIDS virus and thus halts the progression of the disease, it does not cure the patient or reverse existing damage. Patients using zidovudine must continue to take the drug for the rest of their lives in order to prevent the disease from progressing further. They live in a state of AIDS-related limbo in which they neither recover from the disease nor decline significantly in their condition.

Unfortunately, zidovudine is highly toxic and can produce significant side effects in many patients. For this reason, the Food and Drug Administration has approved its use only for a limited range of AIDS victims. Economic factors also prohibit the use of the drug for some AIDS patients who could otherwise potentially receive its benefits. Prescription costs for zidovudine typically run into several thousand dollars per year and payment for this treatment is often excluded from insurance policies and other health care financing programs. AIDS patients who take zidovudine will definitely prolong their lives, but they will do so at great personal expense.

Other AIDS Therapies

The search continues for other therapies that will be effective in treating AIDS patients. While researchers have identified several such candidates, none has been demonstrated to be as effective as zidovudine. Several drugs, including ampligen, AL-721, and dextran sulfate, have been in high demand by AIDS patients, but none of these drugs has been effective in clinical trials. Several genetically-engineered drugs based on various proteins found on the surface of the AIDS virus are being tested, but these therapies have not been as successful as had initially been hoped. In addition to drug therapies, nutrition and other "natural" therapies give hope that the disease can be stopped through a combination of drugs and changes in health-related behavior.

Most of the news surrounding developments in AIDS therapies during 1988 was political rather than medical. AIDS victims and several AIDS-related organizations have long been pressuring the Food and Drug Administration to release potential AIDS drugs more rapidly. While the government has instituted measures to speed the approval of drugs for life-threatening diseases (particularly AIDS), the Food and Drug

Administration also does not want to release drugs to the public that could later be identified as harmful. This issue is further complicated by the fact that many of the experimental AIDS drugs in question are currently in use in other nations that do not require as strict regulations for drug approval.

After much debate, the Food and Drug Administration has now decided to allow individual AIDS victims to import experimental therapies from other nations for their own personal use. This policy allows dying AIDS victims to receive the potential benefits of these experimental new drugs and also allows the government to continue testing new drugs to determine if they have any damaging side effects. While this decision has been applauded by AIDS victims, it is causing some problems for AIDS researchers. Scientists conducting clinical trials of potential AIDS therapies may have their data clouded by the simultaneous use of one or several other therapies followed by the patient without the researcher's knowledge. This policy may help AIDS victims in the short term, but it may actually hinder long-term AIDS drug research.

The Search for a Vaccine

Initial hopes for the early discovery of an AIDS vaccine have vanished. Several vaccines are currently undergoing clinical trials, but many years of testing must be conducted before a vaccine can be released to the public. Several vaccine strategies are currently being tested, including some that are based on genetically engineered proteins found on the AIDS virus. Researchers hope that the virus will bind to these proteins and not to the T-cells of the immune system. If successful, these genetically engineered proteins will prevent the virus from reproducing and thus prevent the onset of AIDS. Although tests of these theories have been successfully completed in the laboratory, complications have arisen during human trials. Researchers fear that vaccines based on the live virus will actually spread the disease rather than prevent it. The genetic variability of the virus is also causing problems for vaccine research. While scientists may develop a vaccine that prevents infection from one strain of the virus, the patient may still become infected by other variations. Researchers are still a long way from developing an effective, accurate, and safe AIDS vaccine.

Transmission of the Virus

Much progress has been made in better understanding the methods of transmission of the AIDS virus. Contaminated blood or blood products, sexual transmission, and transmission from mother to child during pregnancy remain the only pathways for becoming infected by the virus. AIDS is definitely not transmitted by insects, animals, saliva, perspiration, tears, toilet seats, or any other form of casual contact. Persons who do not engage in sexual activities with an infected individual and who do not come into contact with contaminated blood will not become infected by the AIDS virus.

AIDS Among Intravenous Drug Users

Intravenous drug users comprise the group most at risk for AIDS infection. Intravenous drug users frequently share needles and other drug paraphernalia, placing them at a high risk for coming into contact with contaminated blood. The underground nature of this usually illegal activity results in a series of behaviors that enhance the risk of infection. In addition to the risk from needle sharing, drug users are much less likely than other groups to engage in safe sexual practices. The greatest number of cases of heterosexual transmission occur among sexual partners of intravenous drug users. The connection between AIDS and intravenous drug abuse also represents a significant threat to members of minority groups due to the disproportionately high numbers of Blacks and Hispanics who engage in drug abuse.

Heterosexual Transmission of the Virus

Sexual transmission of the AIDS virus is currently the most prevalent form of AIDS transmission in the United States. Sexual transmission applies to both homosexuals and heterosexuals, although the risk to heterosexuals is much less severe than had previously been estimated. The heterosexual epidemic has not occurred due to several factors. The virus is transmitted much more effectively by men than by women. This relatively one-directional transmission vector explains the greater devastation among male homosexuals than among heterosexuals. AIDS education efforts have also been successful in changing the behaviors of many heterosexuals. Condom usage has increased dramatically and heterosexuals are practicing more safe sex when the immune status of their sexual partners is not known.

The most important factor in preventing heterosexual transmission of AIDS is the selection of a sexual partner. As long as an individual does not engage in sex with a person who has AIDS or is known to be infected, the risk of infection is minimal. Continued caution in the choice of a partner and the increase in the practice of safe sex will prevent a heterosexual epidemic.

AIDS in Women and Children

Despite the low risk of heterosexual transmission, the number of women with AIDS is continuing to rise. The vast majority of infected women are sexual partners of men with AIDS. The greatest majority of these women are the partners of intravenous drug users or are intravenous drug users themselves. Low-income minority women who are sexual partners of drug users comprise the fastest growing group of female AIDS victims. Education programs must be designed to reach members of this specific population.

As the number of women with AIDS increases, the number of children with AIDS also rises. Although a few children with AIDS contracted the disease through blood transfusions, the majority of children with AIDS became infected before or during birth. The clinical impact of AIDS on children is different than on adults because children's immune systems are not yet fully developed. Although some research has been conducted on the use of zidovudine with children, it is not yet known if this therapy will be successful in this group of AIDS victims. Children with AIDS are frequently members of low-income minority groups and often end up in the care of the state. Additional research on AIDS in children is needed, as well as an increase in the resources for social services for children with AIDS.

Occupational Transmission of the Virus

There is very little danger of transmission of the AIDS virus through occupational exposure, unless an employee engages in a specific activity at risk for the disease. As long as employees do not share needles or engage in sex with a co-worker who has been infected by the AIDS virus, there is very little danger of transmission. Casual contact with an employee who is infected by the AIDS virus will not cause any danger to other employees. Employees with AIDS should be allowed to work as long as they are healthy enough to successfully carry out their responsibilities. This policy has been supported by the United States Supreme Court and more recently has also been endorsed by the Justice Department. Companies should develop AIDS education programs in order to dispel fears about AIDS and to inform their employees of the facts about the disease.

In contrast to persons in other occupations, health care workers do risk infection through occupational exposure. Several cases have been reported of health care workers who became infected through exposure to contaminated blood or other bodily fluids of AIDS victims. The Centers for Disease Control has issued safety regulations for the handling of all bodily fluids of AIDS patients and prescribed protective clothing for performing various activities with AIDS patients. There is very little risk of infection when these safety precautions are followed.

AIDS Education Programs

The only current method for stopping the spread of the AIDS epidemic is by changing behaviors that place an individual at risk for AIDS. AIDS education programs have generally been successful in creating an awareness of the disease, but they have had mixed results in changing specific behaviors. Studies indicate that the general knowledge level about the disease is high, but that most persons are not acting on that knowledge. Among male homosexuals, education programs have been highly successful in reducing the number of new cases of the disease. Studies indicate a dramatic increase in the use of condoms and the following of safe sexual practices in this group. However, education programs aimed at other populations have not been quite as successful. Future AIDS education programs must be aimed at specific populations who are at risk for the disease and must take into account the cultural and social aspects of those target groups. Changing the sexual and drug use behaviors that place individuals at risk for AIDS are the next goals of AIDS education programs.

AIDS and the Insurance Industry

The insurance industry has been severely affected by the AIDS crisis. Insurers foresee paying a large portion of AIDS health care costs and are seeking methods to minimize their economic losses. AIDS treatments are expensive and insurance companies believe that payments for AIDS claims could bankrupt the entire industry. One insurance company has predicted that AIDS claims will cost insurers over $50 billion by the year 2000. Other experts predict that AIDS will never amount to more than 2% of all health care expenditures in the United States. Insurers would like to use AIDS blood tests to screen applicants for policies, but opponents feel this plan will lead to widespread discrimination against members of high risk groups. Some states have passed legislation outlawing blood testing for insurance reasons, but these laws are currently being challenged in the courts. It will remain to be seen if the disease creates an economic nightmare for insurers and if AIDS blood testing will be used to screen applicants for insurance policies.

AIDS and the Media

Slow progress in the war against AIDS has reduced the coverage of the epidemic by the news media. The discovery of the AIDS virus and the development of zidovudine tended to drive past media interest in the disease. Now that progress has slowed, the media no longer has sensational stories to report. Some media experts feel that the public has grown tired of hearing about AIDS and that the discussion of death and disease has resulted in public apathy. Media interest in AIDS will increase once again when a cure or vaccine is discovered.

The Future of the AIDS Epidemic

The number of AIDS cases will climb as those persons who are currently infected develop the disease. Education efforts may be succeeding in slowing the rate of infection, but the death rate will rise for at least several more years. No hope is seen for an immediate cure or vaccine, although research in these areas is making steady progress. Several mathematical models that predict the future of the disease indicate that AIDS will be with us for some years to come, even if a vaccine is discovered today. Only a global effort such as that being conducted by the World Health Organization will prevent AIDS from devastating the populations and economies of many nations. AIDS education efforts that encourage behavioral change and that are aimed at specific populations at risk for the disease are the only current weapons against the further spread of the virus. We can only hope that these efforts are successful.

David A. Tyckoson
Iowa State University
September 1989

AIDS Update: July - December 1988

1.   Barnes, Deborah M. "Gallo Meeting a Mecca for AIDS Researchers." Science, v. 241, September 9, 1988, p. 1287.
     A small meeting initially designed to review the progress of research in an AIDS laboratory has turned into a premier international conference. This meeting, held in the laboratory of Dr. Robert Gallo, is a place for researchers to exchange results and ideas in a less formal environment than that provided by other meetings.

2.   **Batchelor, Walter F. "AIDS 1988." American Psychologist, v. 43, November 1988, pp. 853-858.**
     Understanding the mechanisms of the AIDS virus means overcoming irrational fears of transmission. Understanding the epidemiology of AIDS is vital to overcoming the prejudice against individuals at risk. Scientists are limited by their own perceptions of the disease.

3.   **Baum, Rudy M. "Tackling AIDS: Scientists Brace for the Difficult Road Ahead." Chemical and Engineering News, v. 66, July 11, 1988, pp. 7-14.**
     A large amount of information has been learned about AIDS in a very short time. The next chapter in the history of AIDS will involve the discovery of an effective therapy or vaccine. Some of the results presented at the Fourth International Conference on AIDS are discussed.

4.   Bazell, Robert. "AIDS Again." New Republic, v. 199, July 18, 1988, pp. 15-16.
     The rate of infection by the AIDS virus is slowing among some groups, but the number of cases of the disease is still rising. The Fourth International Conference on AIDS reminds us that we have a long way to go in stopping the spread of this disease.

5.   Benditt, John. "Report From Stockholm." Scientific American, v. 259, August 1988, pp. 14-15.
     A report on the Fourth International Conference on AIDS. No dramatic breakthroughs were reported, but scientists are steadily adding to their knowledge of the disease.

6.   **Gallo, Robert C. and Luc Montagnier. "AIDS in 1989." Scientific American, v. 259, October 1988, pp. 40-48.**
     The story of the discovery of the AIDS virus is recounted by the two men who first isolated it. The origin of the virus and potential research agendas for a therapy or a vaccine are also discussed.

7.   Goldsmith, Marsha F. "December 1 Designated World AIDS Day: Message Is Join the Worldwide Effort." JAMA: Journal of the American Medical Association, v. 260, November 25, 1988, pp. 2969-2970.
     The World Health Organization has designated December 1, 1988 as World AIDS Day, with activities planned around the globe. The purpose of this day is to raise public awareness and knowledge about the disease.

8.   Goldsmith, Marsha F. "Small Scientific Steps Important in Gigantic AIDS Control Mission." JAMA: Journal of the American Medical Association, v. 260, August 19, 1988, pp. 893-894.
     Over 200,000 cases of AIDS have been estimated to have occurred worldwide and ten million people have been infected by the virus. Education programs are still the most effective means for stopping the spread of the disease. More basic research is needed on the lethality of the AIDS virus.

9.   Hirschfield, Robert. "For Life at the Edge of Life." Christianity and Crisis, v. 48, July 4, 1988, pp. 223-225.
     Communities are attempting to provide the necessary services to care for persons with AIDS. AIDS support services in several cities are profiled.

10.   Hovey, Gail. "AIDS: Simple Lessons." Christianity and Crisis, v. 48, July 4, 1988, pp. 219-221.
     The AIDS epidemic has grown to the point at which it has become everyone's problem. The disease affects different populations in different ways. The resources of the church should be used to help stop the spread of AIDS.

11.   Kingman, Sharon. "AIDS Researchers Book Shuttle Place." New Scientist, v. 119, September 29, 1988, p. 37.
     Scientists are using the space shuttle to try to grow a perfect crystal of an enzyme related to the AIDS virus. If successful, the structure of the crystal may be studied. This may result in a new drug that can interfere with the action of the enzyme and the reproduction of the virus.

12.   Margolis, Stephen. "The AIDS Epidemic: Reality Versus Myth." Judicature, v. 72, June/July 1988, pp. 58-62.
     AIDS has been reported in every state, but it is more concentrated in New York, California, Florida, Texas, and New Jersey. The virus destroys the immune system, leaving it open for other infections. The virus is transmitted through sexual contact and contaminated blood or blood products.

13. Moseley, Charles J. "AIDS Update." Editorial Research Reports, v. 2, December 16, 1988, pp. 630-643.
     An overview of the current state of the AIDS epidemic. The rate of infection, existing therapies, vaccine trials, and the economic and political implications of AIDS are all discussed.

14. Moskop, John C.   "AIDS and Public Health."   Death Studies, v. 12, 1988, pp. 417-431.
     AIDS has created a significant problem for the public health officials who are responsible for stopping the spread of the disease. Several public health issues are reviewed, including education, needle exchange programs, screening of the blood supply, AIDS testing programs, and the isolation of AIDS victims.

15. Nelson, Theodore H. "The Checkmate Proposal." Whole Earth Review, no. 59, Summer 1988, pp. 112-114.
     A new method for testing and identifying persons infected by the AIDS virus is suggested. All persons who participate may wear a pendant indicating that they are members of the program, but those who pass an AIDS blood test will wear special pendants that open to verify test results.

16. "Quarterly Report to the Domestic Policy Council on the Prevalence and Rate of Spread of HIV and AIDS: United States." MMWR: Morbidity and Mortality Weekly Report, v. 37, September 16, 1988, pp. 551-554+.
     As of August 29, 1988, 72,024 cases of AIDS had been reported in the United States. A cumulative total of 365,000 cases is projected by 1992. Over one million persons are currently estimated to have been infected. Several national studies will be conducted to determine the level of infection in the general population.

17. "Report of the Second Public Health Service AIDS Prevention and Control Conference." Public Health Reports, v. 103, supplement 1, 1988, pp. 1-109.
     The complete report of the Public Health Service conference on AIDS. All issues related to the disease are discussed, including epidemiology, prevention, therapies, vaccines, psychological consequences of infection, AIDS among drug users, and AIDS in women, children, and minorities.

18. Steel, M. "IVth International AIDS Conference." Lancet, no. 8601, July 2, 1988, pp. 54-55.
     AIDS research has now come of age. No dramatic breakthroughs were announced at the latest AIDS conference. Research is continuing on antiviral drugs and the level of infection is stabilizing in some populations. However, the war against AIDS is far from over.

19. Thomas, Lewis. "AIDS: An Unknown Distance Still to Go." <u>Scientific American</u>, v. 259, October 1988, p. 152.
     A great deal of progress has been made on AIDS in a very short period of time. However, we still need to learn a great deal about antiviral drugs and the action of the immune system.

20. **United States. Congress. House. Committee on Energy and Commerce. Subcommittee on Health and the Environment.** <u>**AIDS Issues (Part 2)**</u>. **Washington, D.C.: Government Printing Office, 1988. 728p. Superintendent of Documents number Y4.En2/3:100-100.**
     The full text of Congressional hearings on several AIDS bills dealing with testing, counselling, confidentiality, and discrimination. Testimony is provided from several medical and professional associations.

21. **United States. National Library of Medicine.** <u>**AIDS Bibliography**</u>. **Washington, D.C.: Government Printing Office, monthly. 1988-. Superintendent of Documents number HE20.3615/3:vol./no.**
     A bibliography of materials received at the National Library of Medicine relating to AIDS. All citations are derived from the databases created and maintained by the National Library of Medicine, including MEDLINE, CATLINE, AIDSLINE, and CANCERLIT.

Medical and Health Care Aspects of AIDS

22. Adler, Michael W. "Epidemiology of HIV Infection." <u>Journal of the Royal College of Physicians</u>, v. 22, July 1988, pp. 133-135.

   By March 1988, approximately 82,000 cases of AIDS had been reported worldwide. In the United States, the groups with the largest number of cases are homosexual men (64%), intravenous drug users (18%), and homosexual men who are also intravenous drug users (7%). Other high risk groups include hemophiliacs, recipients of blood transfusions, and sexual partners of infected persons.

23. "AIDS-Associated Arthritis." <u>American Family Physician</u>, v. 38, November 1988, p. 295.

   Arthritis has rarely been seen in persons infected by the AIDS virus. Four cases of AIDS patients with subacute arthritis are reported.

24. "AIDS: 1987 Revision of CDC/WHO Case Definition." <u>Bulletin of the World Health Organization</u>, v. 66, 1988, pp. 259-263.

   The clinical definition of AIDS has changed over time as more information has been learned about the disease. The latest changes in the definition of AIDS written by the Centers for Disease Control are presented.

25. Barnes, Deborah M. "AIDS Virus Coat Activates T-Cells." <u>Science</u>, v. 242, October 28, 1988, p. 515.

   The gp120 protein on the envelope of the AIDS virus appears to cause a rise in intracellular calcium levels that causes the T-cells to enter the cell cycle. It is not clear how the virus kills the cells.

26. Barnes, Deborah M. "New Clues About Kaposi's Sarcoma." <u>Science</u>, v. 242, October 21, 1988, pp. 376-377.

   The AIDS virus may trigger the growth of Kaposi's tumors in infected patients. A novel growth factor that is associated with the virus has been linked to Kaposi's sarcoma.

27. Barrick, Bill. "Caring for AIDS Patients: A Challenge You Can Meet." <u>Nursing 88</u>, v. 18, November 1988, pp. 50-60.

   Nurses play an essential role in the care of AIDS patients. Nurses must obtain patient histories, assess the physical condition of the patient, determine the psychological state of the patient, and reduce anxiety about the disease. Some treatments for specific secondary infections are recommended.

28. Bennett, JoAnne. "Helping People With AIDS Live Well at Home." Nursing Clinics of North America, v. 23, December 1988, pp. 731-748.
Home health care is one of the best options for the treatment of AIDS patients. The ability to stay at home enhances the quality of life, increases privacy, and raises the personal dignity of the patient. Nurses who treat AIDS patients in the home environment must be aware of the physical, emotional, and psychological issues related to the disease.

29. Bigbee, Paul D. "Inactivation of Human Immunodeficiency Virus (AIDS Virus) By Gamma X-Ray Irradiation in Body Fluids and Forensic Evidence." FBI Law Enforcement Bulletin, v. 57, July 1988, pp. 8-9.
The AIDS virus can survive in dried strains for several days at room temperature and can survive for over two weeks in liquid bodily fluids. The risk of transmission to forensic investigators is small but real. Radiation may be used to neutralize the virus.

30. "Biologists Appeal Against Cell-Sampling Rule." New Scientist, v. 119, July 21, 1988, p. 37.
The Institute of Biologists is opposed to a government prohibition of studying human cheek tissues in school biology classes. The biologists claim that no risk of transmission of the AIDS virus exists as long as proper safety procedures are followed.

31. Boylston, A. W. and N. D. Francis. "Does It Matter Which Cells Are Infected By the Human Immunodeficiency Virus Type 1?" Journal of Pathology, v. 156, October 1988, pp. 93-96.
The AIDS virus attacks the helper T-cells which express the CD4 antigen. It also infects other cells that have the CD4 antigen. These other infections may occur in the early stages of the disease and may be necessary for the transmission of the virus from one person to another.

32. Clark, Christina et al. "Hospice Care: A Model for Caring for the Person With AIDS." Nursing Clinics of North America, v. 23, December 1988, pp. 851-862.
The hospice philosophy and hospice care are well suited for the treatment of AIDS patients. The use of hospice care for AIDS patients is discussed along with the particular concerns of AIDS patients receiving hospice care.

33. Cotton, Deborah J. "The Impact of AIDS on the Medical Care System." JAMA: Journal of the American Medical Association, v. 260, July 22, 1988, pp. 519-522.
    AIDS has had and will have a tremendous impact on the health care system. Additional personnel will be required to treat patients and to search for a cure. AIDS magnifies existing shortages of key personnel such as nurses and medical technologists. Health care employees are also afraid of becoming infected and often suffer from burnout. Hospitals are devoting more space and resources to AIDS, leaving less for the care of patients with other diseases.

34. Denning, Peter J. "Modeling the AIDS Epidemic." American Scientist, v. 76, November/December 1988, pp. 552-555.
    Mathematical modelling of the AIDS epidemic is important because it can help predict future infection and death rates. Through a workshop of mathematicians and AIDS researchers, the value of this technique has become even more accepted by medical researchers.

35. Duff, Celia and J. Peter Hutchby. "Surveillance of AIDS Cases: How Acceptable Are the Figures?" British Medical Journal. v. 297, October 15, 1988, p. 965.
    A study was made to determine the accuracy of the reporting of AIDS cases. Of nineteen possible cases, seven were unreported and one was reported in a different region of the country than the one in which the patient lived. Reported cases may not represent the true geographic distribution of the disease.

36. Fauci, Anthony S. "The Scientific Agenda for AIDS." Issues in Science and Technology, v. 4, Winter 1988, pp. 33-42.
    The National Institutes of Health research strategy for AIDS must balance creativity with control. The current research agenda covers the areas of epidemiology, the characterization of the virus, the method that the virus uses to destroy the immune system, the development of therapies, and the development of vaccines.

37. Gadsby, Patricia. "The Sugarcoated Virus." Discover, v. 9, July 1988, p. 30.
    The proteins on the outer shell of the AIDS virus have unusually long chains of sugar attached to them. These proteins may cause the antibodies to target the wrong portion of the virus, enabling the virus to survive repeated antibody attacks.

38. Grady, Christine. "HIV: Epidemiology, Immunopathogene-
sis, and Clinical Consequences." Nursing Clinics of North
America, v. 23, December 1988, pp. 683-696.
     Although AIDS is a very new disease, it has already had
a dramatic impact on the world. Scientists have identified
the virus that causes AIDS and are beginning to understand how
it affects the T-cells. The gradual loss of the function of
the immune system leaves the patient open to infection from
other agents, which eventually leads to death.

39. Grady, Denise. "The Shaky Case for an AIDS-Syphilis
Connection." Discover, v. 9, December 1988, pp. 24-25.
     Many cases of persons with syphilis and AIDS have been
reported. Some researchers have even suggested that syphilis
causes AIDS, but this theory has been rejected by most
scientists.

40. Hall, Nicholas R. "The Virology of AIDS." American
Psychologist, v. 43, November 1988, pp. 907-913.
     The AIDS virus attacks and destroys the helper T-cells
that protect the body from infection. It also attacks the
brain directly. Researchers must learn about the activity of
the virus if they are to develop a vaccine or a cure.

41. Harnly, Martha E. et al. "Temporal Trends in the
Incidence of Non-Hodgkin's Lymphoma and Selected Malignancies
in a Population With a High Incidence of Acquired
Immunodeficiency Syndrome (AIDS)." American Journal of
Epidemiology, v. 128, August 1988, pp. 261-267.
     The incidence of Kaposi's sarcoma and other lymphomas
increased significantly among never-married men from 1980 to
1985. These increases correspond to the increase in the
number of cases of AIDS. It is not clear if the rates of
infection will continue to rise.

42. Haseltine, William A. and Flossie Wong-Staal. "The
Molecular Biology of the AIDS Virus." Scientific American,
v. 259, October 1988, pp. 52-62.
     The AIDS virus is highly complicated genetically.
Regulatory genes enable it to remain latent or to reproduce
at various rates. These regulatory factors may provide a clue
to stopping the spread of the virus.

43. Hendricks, Melissa. "AIDS and Antibodies: A Too-Specific
Fit?" Science News, v. 134, July 16, 1988, p. 38.
     By changing only a single amino acid on its surface, the
AIDS virus can avoid detection by its antibodies. This may
explain why different mutations of the virus respond
differently to AIDS antibodies. This also makes the virus
very difficult to control.

44. Hendricks, Melissa. "New Protein Piece for AIDS Puzzle." Science News, v. 134, September 3, 1988, p. 150.
    Two research groups have identified a previously unknown gene of the AIDS virus. A new protein has also been identified that may be able to determine infection status.

45. Henry, Keith. "Setting AIDS Priorities: The Need for a Closer Alliance of Public Health and Clinical Approaches Toward the Control of AIDS." American Journal of Public Health, v. 78, September 1988, pp. 1210-1212.
    Public health programs often overlook the human side of AIDS and clinicians are not always aware of public health issues. Additional studies are needed on the biology of the virus in the genital tract, clinical trials of AIDS drugs need to assess their effectiveness on the genital tract, and health care workers need to implement educational programs to minimize transmission of the virus.

46. Heyward, William L. and James W. Curran. "The Epidemiology of AIDS in the U.S." Scientific American, v. 259, October 1988, pp. 72-81.
    There are currently over 66,000 persons with AIDS in the United States and 300,000 additional cases are expected during the next four years. Risk groups and the geographic distribution of the disease are discussed.

47. "HIV Seroprevalence in Migrant and Seasonal Farmworkers: North Carolina, 1987." MMWR: Morbidity and Mortality Weekly Report, v. 37, September 2, 1988, pp. 517-519.
    Migrant farm workers were screened for infection by the AIDS virus at a clinic in North Carolina. Eleven of 426 blood samples tested positive. Men were twice as likely to be infected as women and Blacks were twice as likely to be infected as members of other racial groups.

48. "Increase in Pneumonia Mortality Among Young Adults and the HIV Epidemic: New York City, United States." MMWR: Morbidity and Mortality Weekly Report, v. 37, September 30, 1988, pp. 593-596.
    The rate of death from pneumonia among young persons has risen dramatically in the last few years, directly corresponding to the increase in the number of cases of AIDS. In New York City, the rate has increased from 4.2 per 100,000 population in 1978 to 19.1 per 100,000 in 1987. Similar increases have been seen in other cities.

49. Kaplan, Jonathan E. et al. "A Six-Year Follow-Up of HIV-Infected Homosexual Men With Lymphadenopathy." JAMA: Journal of the American Medical Association, v. 260, November 11, 1988, pp. 2694-2697.
    Of 75 men with generalized lymphadenopathy identified in 1982 and 1983, 22 had developed AIDS within five years. A sharp decline in the number of helper T-cells was usually associated with the onset of the disease.

50. Katzin, Louise. "CDC Clarifies Universal Precautions." _American Journal of Nursing_, v. 88, October 1988, p. 1322.
      Precautions in handling fluids from AIDS patients do not need to be applied to all bodily fluids. The Centers for Disease Control has established specific guidelines for handling different types of bodily fluids of AIDS victims.

51. King, Michael B. "AIDS and the General Practitioner: Views of Patients With HIV Infection and AIDS." _British Medical Journal_, v. 297, July 16, 1988, pp. 182-184.
      In a recent survey, only one-half of the patients who tested positive for AIDS had informed their physician of that status. Those who did not relay this information feared a negative reaction from the physician and a lack of confidentiality of the information.

52. Kingman, Sharon. "Fresh Clues to the Death of Helper Cells." _New Scientist_, v. 119, September 1, 1988, p. 36.
      The gp120 protein seems to be essential for the T-cells to recognize the AIDS virus. When this protein becomes attached to a T-cell, the infected T-cell is destroyed by others. This process may lead to the eventual loss of all T-cells and the associated immune functions.

53. Kristal, Alan R. et al. "Changes in the Epidemiology of Non-Hodgkin's Lymphoma Associated With Epidemic Human Immunodeficiency Virus (HIV) Infection." _American Journal of Epidemiology_, v. 128, October 1988, pp. 711-718.
      The extent to which AIDS has affected the epidemiology of certain cancers is unknown. The incidence of Kaposi's sarcoma has almost tripled in never-married men aged 25-54. Routinely collected cancer and mortality statistics may be helpful in monitoring the spread of the AIDS epidemic.

54. **Martin, Jeanne P. "Hospice and Home Care for Persons With AIDS/ARC: Meeting the Challenges and Ensuring the Quality."** _Death Studies_, v. 12, 1988, pp. 463-480.
      Home health care is the preferred option in treating AIDS patients when intensive medical care is not necessary. A San Francisco program that provides home care for AIDS patients is profiled. Suggestions are made on providing the best environment for AIDS patients in the home.

55. **Miles, Steven A. "Diagnosis and Staging of HIV Infections."** _American Family Physician_, v. 38, October 1988, pp. 248-256.
      An assessment of the risk of infection by the AIDS virus must be made prior to laboratory testing. Once the diagnosis is made, it is important to determine the precise stage of the disease so that the patient may be appraised about life expectancy and possible therapies.

56. Molgaard, Craig A. et al. "Assessing Alcoholism as a Risk for Acquired Immunodeficiency Syndrome (AIDS)." _Social Sciences and Medicine_, v. 27, 1988, pp. 1147-1152.
   Alcohol abuse is a prominent feature of the homosexual experience and may be considered as a risk factor for AIDS. Alcohol damages the immune system and also reduces the chances that an individual will practice safe sex.

57. Moss, A. R. "Predicting Who Will Progress to AIDS." _British Medical Journal_, v. 297, October 29, 1988, pp. 1067-1068.
   It takes an average of eight to ten years after infection to progress to a full case of AIDS. Four predictors that can be used to determine when the disease will begin are the number of CD4 cells, the presence of the p24 antigen, increased concentrations of beta-2 macroglobulin, and the level of neopterin.

58. "New Nomenclature for HIV Genome Proposed." _Chemical and Engineering News_, v. 66, July 11, 1988, p. 13.
   A proposal has been made to standardize the nomenclature of the genes of the AIDS virus. Because many of these genes were identified by several research groups within a short period of time, several different names currently in use.

59. "Nontuberculosis Mycobacteriosis and Tuberculosis in AIDS." _American Family Physician_, v. 38, September 1988, p. 348.
   Mycobacterial infections are important secondary infections in persons with AIDS. Physicians need to distinguish between tuberculosis and nontubercular mycobacteriosis in order to effectively treat the patient.

60. **Osmond, Dennis et al. "Time of Exposure and Risk of HIV Infection in Homosexual Partners of Men With AIDS." _American Journal of Public Health_, v. 78, August 1988, pp. 944-948.**
   Of 117 sexual partners of homosexual men with AIDS, 85 tested positive for infection. The greatest risk factors were receptive anal intercourse and a high number of sexual partners. The risk of transmission may be greatest at the time of the onset of the disease.

61. "Prevalence of Human Immunodeficiency Virus Antibody in U.S. Active-Duty Military Personnel, April 1988." _MMWR: Morbidity and Mortality Weekly Report_, v. 37, August 5, 1988, pp. 461-463.
   All active-duty military personnel are screened for infection by the AIDS virus. Of over 1.7 million persons who have been tested, 2,232 were infected. Rates of infection are much higher for men than for women and are higher among Blacks and Hispanics than among other racial groups. The rate of infection of military personnel is lower than the general population because members of high-risk groups are under-represented in military service.

62. "Recommendations for Diagnosing and Treating Syphilis in HIV-Infected Patients." MMWR: Morbidity and Mortality Weekly Report, v. 37, October 7, 1988, pp. 600-608.
     The clinical manifestations of syphilis may be altered in a patient with AIDS. Several recommendations and guidelines are presented for diagnosing and treating syphilis in AIDS patients.

63. Redfield, Robert R. and Donald S. Burke. "HIV Infection: The Clinical Picture." Scientific American, v. 259, October 1988, pp. 90-98.
     AIDS is the final manifestation of an immune system disorder that may remain dormant for many years. The virus destroys the helper T-cells, leaving the body open for infection from other agents.

64. Resler, Susan S. "Nutrition Care of AIDS Patients." Journal of the American Dietetic Association, v. 88, July 1988, pp. 828-832.
     Weight loss and depletion are common nutritional complications of AIDS. Maintaining a good nutritional status may help fight secondary infections. Home and community care facilities require nutritional expertise when treating AIDS patients.

65. "Revision of CDC/WHO Case Definition for Acquired Immunodeficiency Syndrome (AIDS)." Bulletin of the Pan American Health Organization, v. 22, 1988, pp. 195-201.
     The clinical and laboratory definition of AIDS has changed over time as new information has become available. The latest case definitions used by the Centers for Disease Control are detailed.

66. Rosenthal, Yukiko and Susan Haneiwich. "Nursing Management of Adults in the Hospital." Nursing Clinics of North America, v. 23, December 1988, pp. 707-718.
     Nurses play a significant role in the care of AIDS patients in the hospital environment. Nurses must be aware of the physical, psychological, emotional, and spiritual needs of the patient. By making an initial assessment, developing diagnoses, implementing treatments, and continually reassessing the needs of the victim, the nurse can offer optimal care to the patient.

67. Safyer, A. W. and Karotkin G. Spies. "The Biology of AIDS." Health and Social Work, v. 13, Fall 1988, pp. 251-258.
     The biological actions of the AIDS virus and the immune system must be understood if social workers are to effectively treat AIDS victims. The biology of the virus and the disease are reviewed.

68. Schofferman, Jerome. "Care of the AIDS Patient." Death Studies, v. 12, 1988, pp. 433-449.
Treatment of AIDS patients requires attention to the biological, psychological, and social aspects of the disease. Treatments are recommended for some of the infections commonly seen in AIDS patients. Too often AIDS patients die without adequate care, housing, and financial resources.

69. Senz, Laurie. "Saliva Inhibits Virus." American Health, v. 7, September 1988, pp. 36-38.
Human saliva contains agents that prevent the AIDS virus from infecting immune system cells. This explains why the virus is not transmitted through kissing.

70. Simonsen, J. Neil et al. "Human Immunodeficiency Virus Infection Among Men With Sexually Transmitted Diseases: Experience From a Center in Africa." New England Journal of Medicine, v. 319, August 4, 1988, pp. 274-278.
Of 340 African men studied, 11.2% tested positive for the AIDS virus. Travel, contact with prostitutes, an intact foreskin, and a history of genital ulcers all correlated positively with infection. Genital ulcers may increase susceptibility to infection.

71. Smiley, M. Lynn. "HIV Infection and AIDS: Definition and Classification of Disease." Death Studies, v. 12, 1988, pp. 399-415.
Infection by the AIDS virus can lead to a wide range of clinical manifestations, from no symptoms at all to a full case of AIDS. A system has been developed to classify the various stages of the disease. The use of a classification system helps researchers understand the progression of the disease more clearly.

72. Stamm, Walter E. et al. "The Association Between Genital Ulcer Disease and Acquisition of HIV Infection in Homosexual Men." JAMA: Journal of the American Medical Association, v. 260, September 9, 1988, pp. 1429-1433.
The association between herpes simplex, syphilis, and AIDS was studied in 200 homosexual men. A positive correlation was found between AIDS infection and past infection by these two sexually transmitted diseases. Efforts aimed at stopping the spread of these two infections may also help stop the spread of AIDS.

73. Streicher, Howard Z. and Emmanuel Heller. "Human Retroviruses and Human Disease." Death Studies, v. 12, 1988, pp. 381-397.
The unique biological properties of retroviruses are essential in understanding their role in causing disease. This has become even more critical since the discovery that one of the viruses in this classification causes AIDS.

74. Sullivan, Patrick. "FPs Have Important Role to Play in AIDS Battle, Ottawa Specialist Says." Canadian Medical Association Journal, v. 139, December 1, 1988, pp. 1092-1093.
     Family physicians must play a greater role in treating AIDS patients. Since they are on the front lines of the health care system, physicians must be able to diagnose and counsel patients who have become infected. They must also reassure those patients who are not infected.

75. "Transmission of HIV Through Bone Transplantation: Case Report and Public Health Recommendations." MMWR: Morbidity and Mortality Weekly Report, v. 37, October 7, 1988, pp. 597-599.
     A case has been reported in which a patient became infected by the AIDS virus during a bone transplant. The use of bone grafts from the patient's own skeletal system will eliminate any possible transmission of the virus in this manner.

76. Ungvarski, Peter. "Assessment: The Key to Nursing an AIDS Patient." RN, v. 51, September 1988, pp. 28-33.
     A complete medical and sexual history is needed to help determine if a patient is at risk for AIDS. Patients who are not at risk need education about the disease and those who are at risk must be counselled about the AIDS blood test. All symptoms of AIDS should be assessed in any patients who test positive for infection by the virus.

77. Ungvarski, Peter. "Coping With Infections That AIDS Patients Develop." RN, v. 51, November 1988, pp. 53-58.
     Patients with AIDS are subject to a wide range of secondary infections. The symptoms and available treatments for several common infections are described. Nurses must take precautions to protect themselves from infection through occupational exposure to the AIDS virus.

78. Valdiserri, Ronald O., Geraldine M. Tama, and Monto Ho. "A Survey of AIDS Patients Regarding Their Experiences With Physicians." Journal of Medical Education, v. 63, September 1988, pp. 726-728.
     A survey was conducted among 45 men with AIDS. The majority (63%) felt that their doctor had accurate medical information about AIDS and 81% felt that their doctor knew about experimental therapies. Less than one-half of the physicians recommended that the patient's sexual partners be tested for AIDS or offered to provide them with education or counselling.

79. Weber, Jonathan N. and Robin A. Weiss. "HIV Infection: The Cellular Picture." Scientific American, v. 259, October 1988, pp. 100-109.
    The AIDS virus attacks cells by binding to the CD4 receptor. It is not entirely clear how the virus injects its own genetic material into a cell. Knowledge of the binding and reproduction of the virus may lead to methods to prevent or stop infection.

80. Weiss, Rick. "HIV: More Tricks Up Its Sleeve." Science News, v. 134, October 15, 1988, p. 244.
    Two new studies indicate that the AIDS virus may interfere directly with other cells. The virus may be carcinogenic and a specific protein on the virus appears to destroy nerve cells.

81. Weiss, Rick. "Well-Bred Cells: Poor Hosts to Viruses." Science News, v. 134, October 1, 1988, p. 213.
    Using genetic engineering, scientists have been able to modify the DNA of mammalian cells to stop the reproduction of a virus within those cells. This technique could possibly be used to stop the reproduction of the AIDS virus within the body.

82. Wilkes, Michael S. et al. "Value of Necropsy in Acquired Immunodeficiency Syndrome." Lancet, no. 8602, July 9, 1988, pp. 85-88.
    Over 100 adult AIDS patients were clinically examined following their deaths. These analyses identified several infections that had not been diagnosed earlier. Most prevalent of these were cytomegalovirus, systemic fungal infection, Kaposi's sarcoma, mycobacterium avium intracellulare, and herpes.

AIDS, Blood Transfusions, and the Blood Supply

83. Cleary, Paul D. et al. "Sociodemographic and Behavioral Characteristics of HIV Antibody-Positive Blood Donors." <u>American Journal of Public Health</u>, v. 78, August 1988, pp. 953-957.

    A study was conducted on 173 blood donors who tested positive for infection from the AIDS virus. Most were young, unmarried males who had identifiable major risk factors. However, 20% of all donors testing positive were women.

84. Giesecke, Johan et al. "Incidence of Symptoms and AIDS in 146 Swedish Haemophiliacs and Blood Transfusion Recipients Infected with Human Immunodeficiency Virus." <u>British Medical Journal</u>, v. 297, July 9, 1988, pp. 99-102.

    The time from AIDS infection to the onset of clinical symptoms was measured in hemophiliacs and blood transfusion recipients. Half of all patients developed symptoms within five to six years.

85. Gregario, David I. and Jeanne V. Linden. "Screening Prospective Blood Donors for AIDS Risk Factors: Will Sufficient Donors Be Found?" <u>American Journal of Public Health</u>, v. 78, November 1988, pp. 1468-1471.

    From 14% to 19% of American males between the ages of 17-75 have personal histories placing them at risk for infection from the AIDS virus. An additional 2% of adult women are also in the high risk category. These numbers are not high enough to cause any reduction in the amount of blood available through the blood supply.

86. Marwick, Charles. "Survey: Blood Donations, Transfusions, and AIDS." <u>JAMA: Journal of the American Medical Association</u>, v. 260, July 15, 1988, pp. 312-314.

    A recent poll indicates that the public believes that it is less likely to contract AIDS through the blood supply than it was five years ago. The poll also indicates that the public is slowly learning that AIDS cannot be transmitted by donating blood. The majority polled felt that criminal penalties should be assessed to those who knowingly donate contaminated blood.

87. Pakkanen, John. "How Safe Is Our Blood Supply?" <u>Reader's Digest</u>, v. 133, July 1988, pp. 37-44.

    Persons who know that they are infected by the AIDS virus should not donate blood. The ELISA blood test identifies most infected blood, but a small amount of contaminated blood does slip through the system. Other AIDS viruses may soon become prevalent, but blood donations are not currently being screened for these viruses.

88. Pakkanen, John. "How Safe Is Our Blood Supply?" <u>Saturday Evening Post</u>, v. 260, September 1988, pp. 50-55.
     Although a few cases of transfusion-associated AIDS are still being reported, the blood supply is generally very safe. Infected persons are asked not to donate blood and the ELISA blood test identifies the vast majority of contaminated blood that is donated.

89. Sandmaier, Marian. "Bank Your Blood?" <u>Mademoiselle</u>, v. 94, September 1988, p. 140.
     Fear of AIDS has led some people to store their own blood for possible future use. The Red Cross does not believe that this is necessary. The blood supply is quite safe and storing blood for a specific person can be very expensive.

AIDS and Hemophiliacs

90. Coles, Peter. "Renewed Efforts By French Hemophiliacs on Compensation." Nature, v. 334, July 14, 1988, p. 94.

The French Hemophiliac Association is seeking compensation for members who contracted AIDS through blood transfusions. At least 226 people were infected before the beginning of blood screening programs.

91. "HIV Transmission By Seropositive Hemophiliacs." American Family Physician, v. 38, October 1988, p. 327.

A study was conducted to determine the transmission of the AIDS virus by hemophiliacs. No nonsexual contacts of this population tested positive, adding further evidence that the virus is not transmitted through casual contact.

92. Jackson, J. B. et al. "Hemophiliacs With HIV Antibody Are Actively Infected." JAMA: Journal of the American Medical Association, v. 260, October 21, 1988, pp. 2236-2239.

A study was conducted to determine if hemophiliacs who tested positive for AIDS infection were in fact infected or if they had only developed antibodies to the virus. Only one of 56 persons in the study did not test positive for the virus itself. It is concluded that positive antibody test results indicate actual infection and not just acquired antibodies.

93. Jason, Janine M. et al. "Human Immunodeficiency Virus Infection in Hemophilic Children." Pediatrics, v. 82, October 1988, pp. 565-570.

Children with hemophilia-associated AIDS tend to be older than other children with AIDS, but they show the same rate of infection by pneumocystis carinii pneumonia and have the same rate of fatality. Hemophilic adults with AIDS demonstrate a much lower pneumocystis infection rate, although the fatality rate from this infection is similar to that in other adults with AIDS.

94. Mason, Patrick J., Roberta A. Olson, and Kathy L. Parish. "AIDS, Hemophilia, and Prevention Efforts Within a Comprehensive Care Program." American Psychologist, v. 43, November 1988, pp. 971-976.

Approximately 92% of the persons with hemophilia A in the United States have been exposed to the AIDS virus. Comprehensive care programs have made rapid and substantive changes in response to AIDS.

95. "Safety of Therapeutic Products Used for Hemophilia Patients." MMWR: Morbidity and Mortality Weekly Report, v. 37, July 29, 1988, pp. 441-444+.
    Hemophiliacs are at a high risk for AIDS infection because they rely on pooled blood products, but this risk has been significantly reduced since the advent of heat treating. Only eighteen patients have become infected since heat treating began and the vast majority of these persons used products that were made by a single manufacturing process. In general, blood products are quite safe.

AIDS and Intravenous Drug Abusers

96. "Amsterdam Targets Its Drug Users." New Scientist, v. 119, August 18, 1988, p. 27.
    Dutch officials are worried about AIDS among drug users, almost one-third of whom are already infected. Needle exchange and methadone maintenance programs are offered to anyone who desires such a program. A liberal attitude toward drugs and sex may make the control of AIDS easier in the Netherlands than in other nations.

97. Ball, John C. et al. "Reducing the Risk of AIDS Through Methadone Maintenance Treatment." Journal of Health and Social Behavior, v. 29, September 1988, pp. 214-226.
    A methadone maintenance program appears to have reduced the risk of AIDS in intravenous drug users. However, 82% of the individuals in the study reverted to intravenous drug use when they left the program. Methadone maintenance reduces the risk for AIDS temporarily, but other treatments or programs are needed to stop the risk completely.

98. **Battjes, Robert J. and Roy W. Pickens. Needle Sharing Among Intravenous Drug Abusers: National and International Perspectives. Washington, D.C.: Government Printing Office, 1988. 183p. National Institute on Drug Abuse Research Monograph number 80. Superintendent of Documents number HE20.8216:80.**
    AIDS presents a significant risk for intravenous drug abusers who share needles and other drug equipment. This document provides the results of a conference on needle sharing, with particular reference to practices among different populations of drug users and possible education programs that can be used to prevent the spread of the AIDS virus.

99. Birchard, Karen. "While Irish Consider How to Limit Spread." New Scientist, v. 120, October 8, 1988, p. 23.
    Researchers in Ireland are looking for ways to stop the spread of AIDS among drug users. Drug users comprise the largest population of infected persons in that nation. The main thrust of the Irish program is to use methadone to bring drug users into counselling programs.

100. **Des Jarlais, Don C. and Samuel R. Friedman. "The Psychology of Preventing AIDS Among Intravenous Drug Users." American Psychologist, v. 43, November 1988, pp. 865-870.**
    Studies of programs to reduce the risk for AIDS among drug users have all reported a decrease in high risk behavior. Successful programs designed to change high risk behaviors must generate motivation for change, provide a means for changing behavior, and reward new behaviors.

101. "Experiment Worth Trying." Commonweal, v. 115, December 2, 1988, p. 645.

  AIDS is growing rapidly among children, who usually contract the disease from their mothers. A needle-exchange program may help prevent the disease from spreading among drug users, who are most at risk for having children with AIDS.

102. Fackelmann, Kathy A. "AIDS Toll Underestimated in IV Drug Users." Science News, v. 134, November 12, 1988, p. 311.

  Statistics on the deaths of drug users in New York City have underestimated the number related to AIDS by as much as one-half. Many drug abusers have died of other diseases that struck them after AIDS had already destroyed their immune systems.

103. Farid, B. T. "AIDS and Drug Addiction Needle Exchange Schemes: A Step in the Dark." Journal of the Royal Society of Medicine, v. 81, July 1988, pp. 375-376.

  Intravenous drug abusers account for 16% of all British cases of AIDS. Needle-exchange programs have been promoted as a means to stop the spread of the disease in this population. This sends a mixed message to drug users, telling them not to use drugs while simultaneously providing them with the materials to do so.

104. Griffin, Glen C. "Free Needles for Addicts?" Postgraduate Medicine, v. 84, August 1988, pp. 15-20.

  Rather than providing free needles to intravenous drug abusers, we should adopt a policy of zero tolerance for illicit drugs. Other methods of stopping the spread of AIDS should be examined. A policy promoting free needles implies an acceptance of this illegal activity.

105. "New Money Heralds Hope for Drug Users." New Scientist, v. 120, October 8, 1988, p. 23.

  The British government is encouraging local health officials to establish needle exchange programs for drug users. This policy follows evidence that drug users are willing to change their drug behaviors to avoid contracting AIDS.

106. "Panacea in Needle Park." U.S. News and World Report, v. 105, November 21, 1988, p. 18.

  In a pilot project designed to stop the spread of AIDS, free needles will be distributed to intravenous drug users in New York City. If this project proves successful, the program may be expanded to include a larger number of drug users.

107. Raymond, Chris A. "Study of IV Drug Users and AIDS Finds Differing Infection Rate, Risk Behaviors." <u>JAMA: Journal of the American Medical Association</u>, v. 260, December 2, 1988, p. 3105.

A Chicago program aimed at preventing the spread of AIDS among drug users has found a wide variation in infection rates within the city. This program uses street contacts to reach those persons that other programs do not treat. It also believes that this street approach may be more effective in educating this population about AIDS.

108. Raymond, Chris A. "U.S. Cities Struggle to Implement Needle Exchanges Despite Apparent Success in European Cities." <u>JAMA: Journal of the American Medical Association</u>, v. 260, November 11, 1988, pp. 2620-2621.

Needle exchange programs have been suggested as a means to prevent the spread of AIDS among drug users, but they have always run into political opposition. Two cities are beginning pilot projects to determine the effectiveness of such programs.

109. Schuster, Charles R. "A Federal Agency Perspective on AIDS." <u>American Psychologist</u>, v. 43, November 1988, pp. 846-848.

AIDS prevention depends on changing behaviors to lessen the risk of infection. Several programs have been developed to encourage intravenous drug abusers to reduce their risk for AIDS. Stopping drug use completely is the highest priority of these programs.

110. Stoneburner, Rand L. et al. "A Larger Spectrum of Severe HIV-1-Related Disease in Intravenous Drug Users in New York City." <u>Science</u>, v. 242, November 11, 1988, pp. 916-919.

An increase in the death rate of intravenous drug users has occurred in New York City. This increase corresponds directly to the rise of the AIDS epidemic. There appears to be a causal relationship between death and AIDS infection. There may be a large underestimation of the impact of AIDS on drug users, Blacks, and Hispanics.

111. Westler, Jean A. <u>Drugs and AIDS: Getting the Message Out</u>. Washington, D.C.: Government Printing Office, 1988. 16p. Superintendent of Documents number HE20.8208:Ac7/3.

A guide to developing AIDS education programs aimed at drug users. Information is provided on planning and presenting the program, involving local media, and using national resources.

112. Zimmerman, David R. "The Engineer's Role in Halting AIDS." <u>Technology Review</u>, v. 91, October 1988, pp. 22-23.

Hypodermic needles are the narrowest and most effective pathway for spreading AIDS. We need to develop needles that can only be used once in order to stop the practice of re-using and sharing needles among drug users.

Screening for Infection and the AIDS Blood Test

113. Ackerman, Sandra. "Testing the AIDS Tests." <u>American Scientist</u>, v. 76, July/August 1988, pp. 344-345.

The first AIDS blood tests to be developed were the ELISA and the Western Blot. These tests are inexpensive to conduct, but have a high rate of false positive results. More accurate tests are being developed, but the HIV-2 virus may not be identified by any of the existing tests. Home test kits will not be permitted in the near future.

114. "AIDS Tests Examined." <u>Economist</u>, v. 308, July 2, 1988, pp. 70-71.

No single test can absolutely determine infection by the AIDS virus. Two tests are currently used in tandem: the ELISA and the Western Blot. These tests are not reliable for populations with a low rate of infection because they have a high rate of false positive results.

115. Burke, Donald S. et al. "Measurement of the False Positive Rate in a Program for Human Immunodeficiency Virus Infections." <u>New England Journal of Medicine</u>, v. 319, October 13, 1988, pp. 961-964.

The false positive rate of AIDS blood tests was studied among civilian applicants for military service. Only one false positive was discovered among 135,187 applicants. A good screening program can produce an acceptable false positive rate.

116. Cates, Willard, Jr. "HIV Counseling and Testing: Does It Work?" <u>American Journal of Public Health</u>, v. 78, December 1988, pp. 1533-1534.

It appears that knowledge of infection by the AIDS virus corresponds to changes in behavior at risk for transmission of the virus. Testing should be encouraged for anyone who is afraid that they may have been exposed to the virus.

117. Coates, Thomas J. "AIDS Antibody Testing." <u>American Psychologist</u>, v. 43, November 1988, pp. 859-864.

The focus of much AIDS activity has been on testing. Changing behaviors will be much more effective in stopping the spread of AIDS than testing. Provisions must be made to counsel and care for persons who test positive for AIDS infection.

118. Connor, Steve. "Health Officers Altered Data on AIDS Test." <u>New Scientist</u>, v. 119, July 14, 1988, p. 34.

A British government laboratory has been accused of altering data in a test of a new AIDS blood test. Two reports issued by the lab indicated differing levels of false positive results, with the final report stating that the test was much less sensitive than the tests indicated.

119. Corcoran, Elizabeth. "Testing Sales." <u>Scientific American</u>, v. 259, August 1988, p. 98.
DNA probes are pieces of DNA that exactly match the genetic sequence of a particular virus. These probes unequivocally identify infection by that virus. If a probe for the AIDS virus is developed, the sales for this industry could improve dramatically.

120. Dagani, Ron. "FDA Approves Five-Minute AIDS Test." <u>Chemical and Engineering News</u>, v. 66, December 19, 1988, p. 5.
A new blood test has been developed that can detect AIDS antibodies in a single drop of blood. This test uses a genetically engineered protein from the AIDS virus. It produces results quickly and is inexpensive to operate.

121. Dyer, Clare. "HIV Testing: BMA Consensus Reached." <u>British Medical Journal</u>, v. 297, July 16, 1988, pp. 161-162.
The British Medical Association has reached a compromise on AIDS blood testing. Testing should only be done on clinical grounds and with the consent of the patient. It is up to the physician to determine how much information derived from the test should be released to the patient.

122. Evengard, B. et al. "Filter Paper Sampling of Blood Infected With HIV: Effect of Heat on Antibody Activity and Viral Infectivity." <u>British Medical Journal</u>, v. 297, November 5, 1988, p. 1178.
A new technique has been established for conducting an AIDS blood test. By using dried filter paper, there is less trauma for the patient and there is no risk of accidental transmission of the virus to health care workers.

123. Ezzell, Carol. "AIDS Test for One-in-Three Newborns." <u>Nature</u>, v. 335, September 1, 1988, p. 7.
A new program has begun that will test one-third of all newborn babies in the United States for infection by the AIDS virus. The purpose of this study is to determine the infection rate of AIDS in the general population.

124. Findlay, Steven. "Speedier New Tests for the AIDS Virus." <u>U.S. News and World Report</u>, v. 105, November 28, 1988, pp. 79-80.
Two new AIDS tests have been developed that provide more rapid results than the existing procedures. One test identifies the AIDS virus rather than its antibodies and is also able to identify recently infected individuals. Public health officials fear that the availability of rapid, inexpensive tests will lead to further discrimination against those who test positive.

125. **Frank, John W. et al.** **"Testing for HIV Infection: Ethical Considerations Revisited."** Canadian Medical Association Journal, v. 139, August 15, 1988, pp. 287-289.
   AIDS testing is both complex and controversial. Knowledge of one's antibody status will not necessarily result in a change of behavior. False-positive readings will cause unnecessary psychological problems, particularly in groups at low risk for infection. Care must be taken to counsel patients before testing is conducted.

126. Goldsmith, Marsha F. "HIV Prevalence Data Mount, Patterns Seen Emerging By End of This Year." JAMA: Journal of the American Medical Association, v. 260, October 7, 1988, pp. 1829-1830.
   A pretest of a national survey to determine the extent of AIDS infection will begin soon. This test will use interviews and blood samples from randomly selected households. A larger sample will be tested later if the data appear to be valid. Other testing programs will target newborn babies, patients at sexually transmitted disease clinics, and intravenous drug users.

127. Gould, Donald. "Whose Body Is It Anyway?" New Scientist, v. 120, November 19, 1988, p. 60.
   The British government is trying to outlaw home AIDS blood test kits. People should have the right to test themselves for infection by the AIDS virus as long as the tests are safe and provide reliable results.

128. Haggerty, Alfred G. "AIDS Testing Breakthrough Could Save $40M." National Underwriter (Life, Health, and Financial Services Edition), v. 92, September 26, 1988, pp. 5+.
   A new AIDS test has been developed that uses only a single drop of blood taken from a finger prick. This eliminates the expenses required in drawing, shipping, and storing vials of blood. The cost of an AIDS blood test can be reduced by as much as one-half by using this method.

129. Heyward, William L. and James W. Curran. "Rapid Screening Tests for HIV Infection." JAMA: Journal of the American Medical Association, v. 260, July 22, 1988, p. 542.
   Several AIDS blood tests are currently available, but none is adequate for use in developing nations. Existing tests require a high cost, sophisticated instrumentation, and the need for refrigeration. Tests for use in these nations must be rapid, easy to perform, require very little instrumentation, have a long shelf life at room temperatures, and be inexpensive to administer.

130. Hull, Harry F. et al. "Comparison of HIV-Antibody Prevalence in Patients Consenting to and Declining HIV-Antibody Testing in an STD Clinic." <u>JAMA: Journal of the American Medical Association</u>, v. 260, August 13, 1988, pp. 935-938.

During a three-month test period, 82% of all patients attending a sexually transmitted disease clinic voluntarily elected to be tested for AIDS. Less than 10% of the volunteers tested positive, while 4% of those who refused tested positive. Male patients who refuse testing are the most likely to be at risk and should receive counselling.

131. Jones, David C. "Iowa Requires Consent Form for AIDS Test." <u>National Underwriter (Property, Casualty, and Employee Benefits Edition)</u>, v. 92, August 1, 1988, pp. 4+. Also in <u>National Underwriter (Life, Health, and Financial Services Edition)</u>, v. 92, August 8, 1988, pp. 4+.

Iowa insurers must now acquire a signed consent form before testing applicants for AIDS infection. This form states specifically the nature of the test and identifies who will have access to test results.

132. Joyce, Christopher. "Five-Minute AIDS Test Cleared in U.S." <u>New Scientist</u>, v. 120, December 24, 1988, p. 6.

A five-minute AIDS blood test has been approved for use in the United States. Because false-positive readings do occur, all positive results should be confirmed by another test. This test is intended primarily for use by emergency health care personnel.

133. Kaminski, Mitchell A. and Peter M. Hartmann. "HIV Testing: Issues for the Family Physician." <u>American Family Physician</u>, v. 38, July 1988, pp. 117-122.

Physicians must understand the ramifications of AIDS blood testing and must provide appropriate counselling both before and after testing. The physician must also be prepared to deal with the psychological and social consequences of a positive test result.

134. Katzin, Louise. "PCR: A New Test for HIV." <u>American Journal of Nursing</u>, v. 88, September 1988, p. 1172.

A new AIDS blood test has been developed that uses the technique of gene amplification. This test can detect a single molecule of viral DNA among one million white blood cells.

135. Kleinman, Irwin. "An Examination of HIV Antibody Testing." <u>Canadian Medical Association Journal</u>, v. 139, August 15, 1988, pp. 289-291.

Prevention is the only way to stop the spread of AIDS and testing is our only tool for determining who has been infected. Physicians should encourage patients to be tested for exposure to the virus.

136. Leukefeld, Carl G. "AIDS Counseling and Testing." <u>Health and Social Work</u>, v. 13, Summer 1988, pp. 167-169.
Counseling is necessary both before a patient decides to take an AIDS blood test and after the results are received. Social workers should take a more active role in the counseling of AIDS patients.

137. Lundberg, G. D. "Serological Diagnosis of Human Immunodeficiency Virus Infection By Western Blot Testing." <u>JAMA: Journal of the American Medical Association</u>, v. 260, August 5, 1988, pp. 674-679.
The Western Blot test is currently the most sensitive and specific test for AIDS infection. However, standards are needed to ensure accurate and consistent results. This test should only be performed by laboratories that use optimal reagents and procedures and that possess a high level of technical skill.

138. McGourty, Christine. "British Physicians Brood on HIV Testing and Designer Children." <u>Nature</u>, v. 334, July 14, 1988, p. 94.
Patients should be tested for infection by the AIDS virus only for clinical purposes and only with their consent. Anonymous screening is needed to gather more information about the extent of infection, but should be done only when the tests cannot be traced back to the individual.

139. McMahon, Kathleen M. "The Integration of HIV Testing and Counseling Into Nursing Practice." <u>Nursing Clinics of North America</u>, v. 23, December 1988, pp. 803-821.
Nurses have historically engaged in health promotion and prevention programs. With the onset of the AIDS epidemic, nurses must take the same professional approach to AIDS testing and prevention activities.

140. Newmark, Peter. "U.K. Government Agrees to Anonymous HIV Testing." <u>Nature</u>, v. 336, December 1, 1988, p. 413.
The British government has agreed to begin anonymous AIDS testing. The need for information on the prevalence of infection outweighs the ethical objections to such a program.

141. Ohi, Gen et al. "Notification of HIV Carriers: Possible Effect on Uptake of AIDS Testing." <u>Lancet</u>, no. 8617, October 22, 1988, pp. 947-949.
A study was conducted to determine if legislation requiring the reporting of persons testing positive for antibodies to the AIDS virus would affect an individual's willingness to be tested. This type of legislation is counterproductive because it causes some of the persons most likely to be infected to avoid testing.

142. Quinn, Thomas C. et al. "Rapid Latex Agglutination Assay Using Recombinant Envelope Polypeptide for the Detection of Antibody to the HIV." <u>JAMA: Journal of the American Medical Association</u>, v. 260, July 22, 1988, pp. 510-513.
    Blood transfusions continue to be a major transmission path for the AIDS virus in developing countries, where screening does not always take place. A new test has been developed that may be used easily on-site to screen blood donations. This test may help to reduce the spread of the virus in Africa and the developing nations.

143. Soskolne, Colin L. "Importance of Counselling in HIV Antibody Testing." <u>Canadian Medical Association Journal</u>, v. 139, October 15, 1988, pp. 709-710.
    Many patients may ask their physicians to be tested for infection by the AIDS virus. Physicians can minimize the medical and social impact of infection by counselling patients before and after testing. Physicians must be aware of the limitations of the test and must place the test into its proper context.

144. Swartz, Martha S. "AIDS Testing and Informed Consent." <u>Journal of Health Politics Policy and Law</u>, v. 13, Winter 1988, pp. 607-621.
    Consent should be obtained before all AIDS testing. Testing patients in order to protect health care workers is not justified if standard safety precautions are followed. The rights of the patient should always have the first consideration.

145. "Trends in Human Immunodeficiency Virus Infection Among Civilian Applicants for Military Service: United States, October 1985-March 1988." <u>MMWR: Morbidity and Mortality Weekly Report</u>, v. 37, November 11, 1988, pp. 677-679.
    Military recruits comprise one of the largest segments of the population which undergoes mandatory AIDS testing. The rate of infection over a three year period was seen to be 1.4 per 1,000 applicants. The infection rate has been steadily dropping over the study period.

146. "Truth in Testing." <u>Science News</u>, v. 134, October 15, 1988, p. 244.
    The false-positive rate of AIDS blood tests has created a problem with the screening of groups that have a very low incidence of infection. In a study of applicants for military service from rural counties, only one false positive was found among 135,187 persons tested.

147. United States. Congress. House. Committee on Energy and Commerce. <u>AIDS Counseling and Testing Act of 1988</u>. Washington, D.C.: Government Printing Office, 1988. 85p. Superintendent of Documents number <u>Y1.1/8:100-783</u>.

A report recommending passage of a bill on AIDS blood testing. This bill would establish a $400 million grant program to encourage voluntary testing. It also provides regulations for maintaining the confidentiality of test results.

148. Weiss, Robin and Samuel Thier. "HIV Testing Is the Answer--What's the Question?" <u>New England Journal of Medicine</u>, v. 319, October 13, 1988, pp. 1010-1012.

The fact that a medical test exists does not mean that it should always be used. Since no cure has been found for AIDS, testing should only be done to screen blood products. Testing will not change patient behavior unless such testing is voluntarily initiated by the patient.

Sexual Behaviors at Risk for AIDS

149. Abramson, Paul R. "Sexual Assessment and the Epidemiology of AIDS." Journal of Sex Research, v. 25, August 1988, pp. 323-346.

Based on several mathematical models, three significant sexual parameters have been identified that correlate with AIDS infection. Homosexuality, the practice of anal intercourse, and the selection of sexual partners are the most important sexual risk factors for AIDS infection.

150. Booth, William. "Social Engineers Confront AIDS." Science, v. 242, December 2, 1988, pp. 1237-1238.

Changing human behavior is difficult, especially when confronting behaviors related to sex and drug abuse. It is not clear how to encourage behavioral changes, but they must be changed in order to stop the spread of AIDS. Most people will not change until the disease affects their own lives.

151. Coates, Randall A. et al. "Risk Factors for HIV Infection in Male Sexual Contacts of Men With AIDS Or an AIDS-Related Condition." American Journal of Epidemiology, v. 128, October 1988, pp. 729-739.

Of 246 healthy male sexual contacts of men with AIDS, 144 tested positive for antibodies to the AIDS virus. There was no correlation between the number of partners and infection status. The highest correlations were found in those men who participated in receptive anal intercourse.

152. Coates, Randall A. et al. "Validity of Sexual Histories in a Prospective Study of Male Sexual Contacts of Men With AIDS Or an AIDS-Related Condition." American Journal of Epidemiology, v. 128, October 1988, pp. 719-728.

A survey was conducted to determine the sexual practices of homosexual men with AIDS. There seemed to be an excellent correlation between infection and a majority of sexual activities. This data can be used to assess the risk of becoming infected through specific sexual practices.

153. Fisher, Jeffrey D. "Possible Effects of Reference Group-Based Social Influence on AIDS-Risk Behavior and AIDS Prevention." American Psychologist, v. 43, November 1988, pp. 914-920.

Individual behaviors are strongly related to those of other members of their peer reference group. When the behavior of the group includes high-risk activities, individuals will be reluctant to change their own behaviors. Several strategies are provided for promoting AIDS-prevention behaviors to groups at risk.

154. Ishii-Kuntz, Masako. "Acquired Immune Deficiency Syndrome and Sexual Behavior Changes in a College Student Sample." <u>Sociology and Social Research</u>, v. 73, October 1988, pp. 13-18.

The level of concern of college students about AIDS is directly related to their perceived change in sexual behavior. However, increased information about AIDS does not necessarily lead to behavioral changes.

155. Lever, Janet. "Condoms and Collegians." <u>Playboy</u>, v. 35, September 1988, pp. 79-80+.

Many college students do not feel that AIDS will have any affect on them. They are aware of the disease, but have not changed their sexual behaviors to avoid risk of infection.

156. Mangan, Katherine S. "Sexually Active Students Found Failing to Take Precautions Against AIDS." <u>Chronicle of Higher Education</u>, v. 35, September 28, 1988, pp. A1+.

Although AIDS education programs exist in many colleges, most students do not think that they will be affected and have not changed their sexual behaviors to avoid infection. More creative and personal AIDS education programs are needed.

157. "Number of Sex Partners and Potential Risk of Sexual Exposure to Human Immunodeficiency Virus." <u>MMWR: Morbidity and Mortality Weekly Report</u>, v. 37, September 23, 1988, pp. 565-568.

A survey was conducted to determine the number of sexual partners of an average segment of American adults. Over 80% of those who responded indicated that they had one or no sexual partners during the previous year. Only 10% indicated that they had between two and four sexual partners and 2% stated that they had over five sexual partners. Only 9% of the men in the study stated that some of their sexual partners had been other men.

158. "Partner Notification for Preventing Human Immunodeficiency Virus (HIV) Infection: Colorado, Idaho, South Carolina, Virginia." <u>MMWR: Morbidity and Mortality Weekly Report</u>, v 37, July 1, 1988, pp. 393-396+.

Partner notification is used in some states as a means of identifying persons at risk of infection by the AIDS virus. Counselling is offered to all sexual and needle-sharing partners of anyone known to be infected by the AIDS virus. Over 80% of the partners contacted have decided to take the AIDS blood test.

159. Reinisch, June M., Stephanie A. Sanders, and Mary Ziemba-Davis. "The Study of Sexual Behavior in Relation to the Transmission of Human Immunodeficiency Virus." <u>American Psychologist</u>, v. 43, November 1988, pp. 921-927.

In order to promote safe sexual practices for AIDS, we must first obtain a precise understanding of existing human sexual behaviors. Statistical data are presented on a variety of sexual behaviors.

160. Ross, Michael W. "Prevalence of Classes of Risk Behaviors for HIV Infection in a Randomly Selected Australian Population." <u>Journal of Sex Research</u>, v. 25, November 1988, pp. 441-450.

A sample of over 2,600 Australians was surveyed for behaviors at risk for transmission of the AIDS virus. The level of homosexuality and contact with prostitutes were much less frequent than those reported by Kinsey in the United States. The risk of infection for Australians may be lower than that for Americans.

161. Siegel, Karolynn et al. "Patterns of Change in Sexual Behavior Among Gay Men in New York City." <u>Archives of Sexual Behavior</u>, v. 17, December 1988, pp. 481-497.

A survey of 162 asymptomatic homosexual and bisexual men revealed that 84% of the population had shown some behavioral changes related to AIDS. The majority of these changes involved a reduction in the number of sexual partners. However, almost one-half of the men in the study still engaged in some high-risk behaviors.

162. Stall, Ron D., Thomas J. Coates, and Colleen Hoff. "Behavioral Risk Reduction for HIV Infection Among Gay and Bisexual Men." <u>American Psychologist</u>, v. 43, November 1988, pp. 878-885.

AIDS education programs have resulted in one of the most profound periods in history of behavior modification for public health purposes. Changes in the behavior of homosexual and bisexual men are discussed.

163. Van Griensven, Godfried J. P. "Impact of HIV Antibody Testing on Changes in Sexual Behavior Among Homosexual Men in the Netherlands." <u>American Journal of Public Health</u>, v. 78, December 1988, pp. 1575-1577.

In a study of homosexual men in Amsterdam, persons who were aware of their own infection showed a distinct reduction in the number of their sexual partners. These men also showed some changes in their sexual practices.

164. Winkelstein, Warren, Jr. et al. "The San Francisco Men's Health Study: Continued Decline in HIV Seroconversion Rates Among Homosexual/Bisexual Men." <u>American Journal of Public Health</u>, v. 78, November 1988, pp. 1472-1474.

The incidence of AIDS infection has been monitored in a group of men in San Francisco since 1984. A decline in the rate of infection in this group corresponds directly with a reduction in the amount of high-risk behavior.

Heterosexual Transmission of the AIDS Virus

165. "Best AIDS Prevention: Choosing Partner Carefully." <u>American Pharmacy</u>, v. 28, August 1988, pp. 11-12.

The choice of a sexual partner is the single most important factor for the risk of AIDS infection. The risk of infection from one heterosexual encounter with a person who is not a member of a high risk group is estimated to be 1 in 5,000,000.

166. Black, David. "An Era of Indifference." <u>American Health</u>, v. 7, October 1988, pp. 87-88.

AIDS will not become epidemic among heterosexuals. The statistical increase in heterosexual transmission is an aberration and the chances of contracting the disease among middle class, non-drug using heterosexuals is minimal. The media has jumped on this concept in its attempt to regulate our sexual behavior.

167. Ellis, Rosemary. "The Fears and Facts of Sex Now." <u>Glamour</u>, v. 86, July 1988, pp. 154-155.

Some questions on the safety of sex are answered, including those dealing with the risk of becoming infected, the safety of condoms, and when to take an AIDS blood test.

168. Fauci, Anthony S. "How Far Will AIDS Spread in the United States." <u>Futurist</u>, v. 22, July/August 1988, pp. 41-42.

It is likely that the rate of infection in the United States is plateauing, even though the disease rate continues to rise. AIDS will not be a great danger to heterosexuals because the prevalence of infection in this population is very low.

169. Hacinli, Cynthia. "AIDS, Straight: A Heterosexual Risk Update." <u>Mademoiselle</u>, v. 94, August 1988, p. 138.

AIDS is a risk to heterosexuals, but it is not as rampant as some past predictions have indicated. The virus is not spread by kissing and no documented cases of transmission during oral sex have been reported. Condoms are recommended as protection during intercourse.

170. Handsfield, H. H. "Heterosexual Transmission of Human Immunodeficiency Virus." <u>JAMA: Journal of the American Medical Association</u>, v. 260, October 7, 1988, pp. 1943-1944.

Sexual behavior modification must be pursued in order to stop the heterosexual spread of the AIDS virus. The virus is spread much more efficiently from men to women than from women to men. This fact may limit the extent of the heterosexual contribution to the AIDS epidemic.

171. Haverkos, Harry W. and Robert R. Edelman. "The Epidemiology of Acquired Immunodeficiency Syndrome Among Heterosexuals." JAMA: Journal of the American Medical Association, v. 260, October 7, 1988, pp. 1922-1929.
    Evidence of heterosexual transmission of the AIDS virus first appeared in Africa and Haiti. In the United States, 26% of the female and 2% of the male cases have been linked to heterosexual transmission. This number may be underestimated due to restrictions of the case definition of the disease. Some recommendations are made to minimize the risk of heterosexual transmission.

172. Kaplan, Edward H. "Crisis? A Brief Critique of Masters, Johnson, and Kolodny." Journal of Sex Research, v. 25, August 1988, pp. 317-322.
    A report by Masters and Johnson claims that AIDS presents a high risk for heterosexuals. A statistical analysis of their data indicates that the risk to heterosexuals is only 2% that to homosexuals. AIDS will only become epidemic if the average number of sexual partners per person per year increases to at least 5.3.

173. Kreigman, Mitchell. "Kiss Me: The Erotic Possibilities of Safe Sex." Glamour, v. 86, August 1988, p. 300.
    Having to think about AIDS can cause people to lose interest in sex. One man has relearned the sexiness of other activities, particularly kissing.

174. Paalman, M. E. M. "Safer Sex." World Health, November 1988, pp. 14-15.
    Everyone who has had more than one sexual partner since 1980 should practice safe sex. Condoms should be used during intercourse and expressions of intimacy other than intercourse should be encouraged.

175. Petersen, James R. "Unrealistic Fear." Playboy, v. 35, July 1988, pp. 49-51+.
    A new book by the noted sex researchers Masters and Johnson states that AIDS is a threat to the heterosexual community and that the virus may be transmitted through casual contact. Scientists have no evidence to support either of these arguments.

176. Tierney, John. "Straight Talk." Rolling Stone, November 17, 1988, pp. 122-137.
    Although there is a risk to heterosexuals from AIDS, it is much lower than previously estimated. Many of the persons claiming to have become infected through heterosexual transmission actually became infected through other means. The media has tended to exaggerate the heterosexual threat.

177. Van der Ende, Marchina E., Philip Rothbarth, and Jeanne Stibbe. "Heterosexual Transmission of HIV By Hemophiliacs." <u>British Medical Journal</u>, v. 297, October 29, 1988, pp. 1102-1103.

A study was conducted on the heterosexual transmission of the AIDS virus among spouses of thirty-five male hemophiliacs. Seven of the men developed AIDS, but none of the spouses became infected. The risk of heterosexual transmission is estimated to be less than 0.1%.

178. Weber, Bruce. "A Man's Report on His Dwindling Options, the Rewards of Waiting." <u>Glamour</u>, v. 86, July 1988, pp. 152-153.

AIDS has changed the sex life of singles. Casual sex has become a thing of the past and sex has become more meaningful and full of hope.

Women and AIDS

179. Hillard, Paula A. "AIDS and Pregnancy." <u>Parents'</u>
<u>Magazine</u>, v. 63, July 1988, pp. 144-146.

A pregnant woman who tests positive for exposure to the
AIDS virus risks transmitting the virus to her unborn child.
This risk is estimated to be between 20%-50% of all births.
Pregnant women should receive counselling prior to deciding
if they would like to be tested for infection.

**180. "Incidence of Acquired Immune Deficiency Syndrome Among
Women in Canada." <u>Canadian Medical Association Journal</u>, v.
139, November 15, 1988, pp. 939-941.**

Of the 1,918 cases of AIDS that have been reported in
Canada, 98 were women. Of these women, approximately one-
third are immigrants from countries where AIDS is endemic,
one-third are heterosexual partners of infected men, and one-
third are recipients of contaminated blood products. The
number of women with AIDS can be used as a measure of the
heterosexual transmission rate of the disease.

181. "One Woman's Crusade." <u>American Health</u>, v. 7, August
1988, pp. 20-23.

AIDS is the biggest killer of women age 25-34 in New York
City. Women need to form support groups and lobby for AIDS
education programs designed to stop the spread of the disease.

182. Roth, Margaret. "A New Burden for Rape Victims." <u>Ms</u>,
v. 17, August 1988, pp. 81-82.

In addition to the trauma of rape, victims must now worry
about the threat of infection by the AIDS virus. Treatment
for AIDS should only begin if it is determined that the rapist
is infected, but this information is not available without his
consent. It is not clear if blood testing would have a
positive or negative effect on rape victims.

Children and AIDS

183. Boland, Mary G. et al. "Children With HIV Infection: Collaborative Responsibilities of the Child Welfare and Medical Communities." <u>Social Work</u>, v. 33, November/December 1988, pp. 504-509.

As the number of children with AIDS grows, child welfare agencies must find foster homes to care for these victims. The collaborative efforts of the New Jersey Department of Human Services and a private hospital are described.

184. Brooks-Gunn, J., Cherrie B. Boyer, and Karen Hein. "Preventing HIV Infection and AIDS in Children and Adolescents." <u>**American Psychologist**</u>**, v. 43, November 1988, pp. 958-964.**

Over 900 children under thirteen years of age currently have AIDS. Most of these children became infected either before birth or through blood transfusions. Adolescents tend to be at risk for AIDS due to their sexual and drug use behaviors. Education programs aimed at adolescents must incorporate information on sexual behaviors.

185. Brown, Larry K. and Gregory K. Fritz. "Children's Knowledge and Attitudes About AIDS." <u>Journal of the American Academy of Child and Adolescent Psychiatry</u>, v. 27, July 1988, pp. 504-508.

In a survey of seventh and tenth grade students, the majority recognized that AIDS is sexually transmitted. No correlation was seen between knowledge levels and behavior, suggesting that education alone will not reduce the risk for this population.

186. "Clinical Manifestations of HIV Infection in Children." <u>American Family Physician</u>, v. 38, October 1988, pp. 378-380.

AIDS infection is difficult to diagnose in children, especially since many children show no clinical signs of the illness for several years. Some specific indicators of AIDS infection are given.

187. Cooper, Ellen R., Stephen I. Pelton, and Mirielle LeMay. "Acquired Immunodeficiency Syndrome: A New Population of Children at Risk." <u>**Pediatric Clinics of North America**</u>**, v. 35, December 1988, pp. 1365-1387.**

AIDS has been known to occur in children since 1982, but the disease is much harder to detect in children than in adults. The current state of knowledge about AIDS infection in children is presented along with related medical, legal, and psychosocial issues.

188. "Epidemiology, Clinical Features, and Prognostic Factors of Pediatric HIV Infection." Lancet, no. 8619, November 5, 1988, pp. 1043-1045.
     Children born infected by the AIDS virus fared worse than those who became infected at a later age. Severe infections were linked with a high mortality rate in this group. The perinatal infection rate was found to be 32.6%.

189. Eron, Carol. "Children and AIDS." Science News, v. 134, July 30, 1988, p. 72.
     Most children with AIDS become infected during pregnancy. By 1991, 10,000 to 20,000 cases of children with AIDS will occur.

190. Goldsmith, Marsha F. "Stockholm Speakers on Adolescents and AIDS: Catch Them Before They Catch It." JAMA: Journal of the American Medical Association, v. 260, August 12, 1988, pp. 757-758.
     The number of adolescents with AIDS is rising slowly but steadily. This group is especially at risk because they engage in dangerous behaviors and generally have a sense of invulnerability. Education programs must target teenagers and teach them not to participate in high risk sexual and intravenous drug activities.

191. Hermann, Richard C. "Center Provides Approach to Major Social Ill: Homeless Urban Runaways and Throwaways." JAMA: Journal of the American Medical Association, v. 260, July 15, 1988, pp. 311-312.
     Homeless adolescents are at a high risk for AIDS, but are not often reached by standard AIDS education programs. A San Francisco youth center is making a special effort to teach runaway teenagers about AIDS.

192. "HIV Infection, Breastfeeding, and Human Milk Banking." Lancet, no. 8603, July 16, 1988, pp. 143-144.
     The AIDS virus has been isolated from human breast milk. This method of transmission has been implicated in four cases of children with AIDS. The danger of withholding breast milk from children is greater than the risk of transmission of the virus.

193. Katzin, Louise. "Immunizing HIV-Positive Children." American Journal of Nursing, v. 88, October 1988, p. 1322.
     In contrast to previous recommendations, the Centers for Disease Control has stated that all children should receive vaccinations, including those infected by the AIDS virus. The risk of disease in unvaccinated children is greater than the risk from the vaccine.

194. Kemper, Kathi and Brian Forsyth. "Medically Unnecessary Hospital Use in Children Seropositive for Human Immunodeficiency Virus." <u>JAMA: Journal of the American Medical Association</u>, v. 260, October 7, 1988, pp. 1906-1909.

Of 34 children studied in a New Haven hospital, over 50% of all of their combined hospital visits were deemed medically unnecessary. The rate of unnecessary hospital stays has decreased over time with the improvement of outpatient services and with increased access to foster care.

195. Kirkland, Martin and Dean Ginther. "Acquired Immune Deficiency Syndrome in Children: Medical, Legal, and School-Related Issues." <u>School Psychology Review</u>, v. 17, 1988, pp. 304-310.

The medical, biological, legal, psychological, and educational issues of AIDS in school-aged children are presented. Several national guidelines, federal regulations, and legal problems are also discussed.

196. "Management of Children Infected With Human Immunodeficiency Virus." <u>Canadian Medical Association Journal</u>, v. 139, September 1, 1988, pp. 391-392.

The Canadian Pediatric Society has endorsed the recommendations on AIDS issued by the American Academy of Pediatrics. Universal precautions should be taken when handling blood and other bodily fluids of children with AIDS.

197. Miller, Jaclyn and Thomas O. Carlton. "Children and AIDS: A Need to Rethink Child Welfare Practice." <u>Social Work</u>, v. 33, November/December 1988, pp. 553-555.

The number of children born with AIDS is increasing rapidly. Society must prepare itself to deal with this problem by establishing the necessary legal and social services to handle and care for children with AIDS.

198. "Mother-to-Child Transmission of HIV Infection." <u>Lancet</u>, no. 8619, November 5, 1988, pp. 1039-1043.

A follow-up study is being conducted on 271 children of mothers infected by the AIDS virus. After one year, ten had developed AIDS and twenty-two showed some symptoms of the disease. The vertical transmission rate is estimated to be 24%.

199. "Perinatal Human Immunodeficiency Virus Infection." <u>Pediatrics</u>, v. 82, December 1988, pp. 941-944.

The primary risk of AIDS infection in children is from a mother who became infected before or during pregnancy. The risk of infection depends on several factors, but is estimated to range from 30% to 50%. Infection is difficult to measure in infants because antibodies produced by the mother may persist for up to fifteen months.

200. Siegel, Micki. "The Youngest Victims: Children With AIDS." Good Housekeeping, v. 207, August 1988, pp. 106-107+.
A report on several children with AIDS. Many are simply left abandoned in the hospital while others have been refused entry into schools. All have had to face both the disease and its social consequences.

201. United States. Congress. House. Select Committee on Children, Youth, and Families. Continuing Jeopardy: Children and AIDS. Washington, D.C.: Government Printing Office, 1988. 12p. Superintendent of Documents number Y4.C43/2:Ac7/4.
AIDS continues to be a risk for children and adolescents. The care of children with AIDS is stretching the limits of existing health care services. Education programs must be increased and a greater response at the national level is needed.

202. United States. Department of Health and Human Services. Final Report: Secretary's Work Group on Pediatric HIV Infection and Disease. Washington, D.C.: Government Printing Office, November 18, 1988. 92p. Superintendent of Documents number HE1.2:P34.
The number of cases of AIDS among children is constantly growing. As of August 15, 1988, 1,125 cases of AIDS have been reported in children under 13 years of age and 289 additional cases have been reported in children age 13-19. Several recommendations are made for improving the government response to the pediatric AIDS problem.

203. "Vertical Transmission of HIV." Lancet, no. 8619, November 5, 1988, pp. 1057-1058.
As of September 12, 1988, the number of perinatal AIDS cases in the United States had reached 902. This number accounts for 78% of all pediatric cases and 1.2% of the total in all populations. Studies on the rate of perinatal infection have produced a wide range of results.

204. Ward-Wimmer, Dorothy. "Nursing Care of Children With HIV Infection." Nursing Clinics of North America, v. 23, December 1988, pp. 719-729.
AIDS has created an entirely new population of terminally ill children. Issues in the care of such children are highlighted, along with the experiences of the children and their families.

205. "Wholly Innocent." Commonweal, v. 115, December 16, 1988, pp. 675-676.
It is estimated that over 20,000 children will be infected by the AIDS virus by 1991. Most of these children will have become infected before birth. Volunteers are needed to care for these children through foster homes and social services.

206. Windom, Robert E. "From the Assistant Secretary for Health." JAMA: Journal of the American Medical Association, v. 260, July 1, 1988, p. 18.

As of April 1988, 955 cases of AIDS among children had been reported. In over three-fourths of the cases, the virus was transmitted during pregnancy. Physicians and social services must be prepared to care for children with AIDS.

Minority Groups and AIDS

207. Amaro, Hortensia. "Considerations for Prevention of HIV Infection Among Hispanic Women." <u>Psychology of Women Quarterly</u>, v. 12, December 1988, pp. 429-443.

Hispanics are disproportionately affected by the AIDS epidemic. Prevention programs aimed at the Hispanic population must take into account the unique cultural factors that differentiate this population from others.

208. Lester, Calu and Larry L. Saxxon. "AIDS in the Black Community: The Plague, the Politics, the People." <u>**Death Studies**</u>**, v. 12, 1988, pp. 563-571.**

The Black community has denied that AIDS is a problem and has not developed the support services necessary to cope with the disease. Intravenous drug use continues at a high rate in this population and provides an effective pathway for the virus. Blacks must face the problem of AIDS before it escalates even further.

209. Mays, Vickie M. and Susan D. Cochran. "Issues in the Perception of AIDS Risk and Risk Reduction Activities By Black and Hispanic/Latina Women." <u>American Psychologist</u>, v. 43, November 1988, pp. 949-957.

AIDS poses a serious threat to Black and Hispanic women, particularly poor women in areas of a high incidence of AIDS. Many members of this population do not feel that they are at risk for infection. The influence of minority culture on their behavior must be considered when designing AIDS education programs.

210. Padgett, Tim. "Waking Up to a Nightmare." <u>Newsweek</u>**, v. 112, December 5, 1988, pp. 24-29.**

Hispanics account for only 8% of the population of the United States, but they have 15% of all AIDS cases. AIDS is prevalent among Hispanic drug abusers, their sexual partners, and their children. Machismo, homophobia, and sexual taboos combine to make Hispanics a difficult group to target with AIDS programs.

211. Peterson, John L. and Gerardo Marin. "Issues in the Prevention of AIDS Among Black and Hispanic Men." <u>American Psychologist</u>, v. 43, November 1988, pp. 871-877.

Minorities account for nearly 40% of all cases of AIDS in the United States. Homosexual or bisexual behavior and intravenous drug abuse have been linked to the majority of AIDS cases among minority men. Information designed to stop the spread of AIDS in this population must be culturally relevant.

212. Randolph, Laura B. "Ebony Interview With U.S. Surgeon General C. Everett Koop." <u>Ebony</u>, v. 43, September 1988, pp. 154-160.

Black Americans, especially women and children, are among the groups most at risk for AIDS. The Surgeon General discusses the risk of AIDS to the Black community.

213. Ron, Aaron and David E. Rogers. "New York City's Health Care Crisis: AIDS, the Poor, and Limited Resources." <u>JAMA: Journal of the American Medical Association</u>, v. 260, September 9, 1988, p. 1453.

AIDS is overwhelming the health care system in New York City. Most new AIDS cases are related to drug abuse and 80% of the patients are Black or Hispanic. This causes an ethical conflict between caring for poor minorities with AIDS or for middle and upper class whites with other diseases.

214. Selik, Richard, Kenneth G. Castro, and Marguerite Pappaioanou. "Racial/Ethnic Differences in the Risk of AIDS in the United States." <u>American Journal of Public Health</u>, v. 78, December 1988, pp. 1539-1545.

The risk of infection by the AIDS virus among Blacks and Hispanics is highest in the northeast region and is higher in the suburbs than in the central city. Risks are greatest for intravenous drug users and are also high for bisexual males.

Zidovudine as a Therapy for AIDS

215. Campbell, Duncan. "AIDS: Patient Power Puts Research on Trial." <u>New Scientist</u>, v. 120, November 12, 1988, pp. 26-27.

Trials of the drug zidovudine have been plagued by problems. Patients may not agree to a study unless they are assured that they are receiving the drug. Some patients will pool their drugs or will be tested independently to ensure that they are receiving the therapy. Scientists are worried that changes in study design will result in inconsistent and inconclusive data.

216. Creagh-Kirk, T. et al. "Survival Experience Among Patients With AIDS Receiving Zidovudine: Follow-Up of Patients in a Compassionate Plea Program." <u>**JAMA: Journal of the American Medical Association**</u>**, v. 260, November 25, 1988, pp. 3009-3015.**

In a study of 4,805 AIDS patients who had received the drug zidovudine to treat pneumocystis carinii pneumonia infection, 73% of the patients had survived after 44 weeks. Patients with a higher base hemoglobin level had an even higher survival rate. These data support the fact that zidovudine increases the life span of AIDS victims.

217. "Evidence Grows in Favour of AIDS Drug." <u>New Scientist</u>, v. 120, December 3, 1988, p. 24.

There is an increasing body of evidence that the drug zidovudine prolongs the life of persons with AIDS. All tests conducted to date have shown that patients taking the drug have performed much better than the control groups.

218. Katzin, Louise. "Prophylactic Retrovir Study for Health Care Workers." <u>American Journal of Nursing</u>, v. 88, July 1988, pp. 950-951.

A study is being conducted on the use of zidovudine to prevent occupational infection in health care workers. The drug is administered immediately following any accident that might transmit the virus.

219. Patlak, Margie. "The Treatment Dilemma." <u>**Discover**</u>**, v. 9, October 1988, pp. 26-27.**

Zidovudine has been authorized only for use with persons who have a fully developed case of AIDS. This raises the ethical problem of withholding a known therapy from a deserving patient only because that patient shows no symptoms of disease. It is also not clear if children should be treated with zidovudine since it is not known if they are truly infected until many months after birth.

220. Pizzo, Philip A. et al. "Effect of Continuous Intravenous Infusion of Zidovudine (AZT) in Children With Symptomatic HIV Infection." New England Journal of Medicine, v. 319, October 6, 1988, pp. 889-896.
     The drug zidovudine was given continuously to 21 children who had been infected by the AIDS virus. Improvement was found in all 13 children who had exhibited encephalopathy before treatment, as well as in five other children. Continuous administration of zidovudine is beneficial to children with AIDS.

221. Pottage, John C., Jr. et al. "Treatment of Human Immunodeficiency Virus-Related Thrombocytopenia With Zidovudine." JAMA: Journal of the American Medical Association, v. 260, November 25, 1988, pp. 3045-3048.
     The drug zidovudine was used to treat AIDS patients suffering from thrombocytopenia infection in three patients. All three patients showed increased platelet counts and decreases in circulating p24 antigen levels. Further testing is needed to determine if zidovudine is an effective therapy for AIDS patients suffering from this infection.

222. Raloff, Janet. "Surprising Boost for Children With AIDS." Science News, v. 134, October 8, 1988, p. 231.
     Children with AIDS have much more visible brain disease than adults and it is possible that brain damage occurs in all children with AIDS. However, the treatment of children with AIDS with zidovudine creates a dramatic reversal of this condition.

223. Rovner, Julie. "Congress Agrees to Extend AZT Funds for AIDS Victims." Congressional Quarterly Weekly Report, v. 46, October 1, 1988, p. 2714.
     Congress has passed emergency legislation that extends a program to provide zidovudine for AIDS patients. This bill authorizes the spending of $15 million over the next six months.

224. Schmitt, Frederick A. et al. "Neuropsychological Outcome of Zidovudine (AZT) Treatment of Patients With AIDS and AIDS-Related Complex." New England Journal of Medicine, v. 319, December 15, 1988, pp. 1573-1578.
     In a double-blind study of the drug zidovudine and a placebo, patients receiving the drug showed a reduction in stress and an improvement in cognitive function. Some of the neurological problems associated with AIDS may be partially relieved with zidovudine.

The Search for Other AIDS Drugs and Therapies

225. "AIDS Treatment Still Focuses on Zidovudine, But Other Agents Are Being Investigated." <u>Chemical and Engineering News</u>, v. 66, July 11, 1988, pp. 8-9.

Zidovudine remains the primary therapy for treating AIDS victims. Patients taking zidovudine survive longer and show more clinical improvements when compared to other AIDS patients. Research is currently underway on other possible therapeutic agents, including the CD4 protein and dextran sulfate.

226. "Ampligen Proves Less Than Able Against AIDS." <u>New Scientist</u>, v. 120, November 5, 1988, p. 23.

A trial of the drug Ampligen for treating AIDS patients ended early because there was no evidence that the drug was working. This result is surprising, since initial investigations indicated that Ampligen both stimulated the immune system and inhibited the virus.

227. Anderson, Alun and David Swinbanks. "U.S. Protests About Possible Drugs for AIDS Treatment." <u>Nature</u>, v. 334, July 7, 1988, p. 3.

A group of AIDS patients has staged a protest against the Japanese manufacturer of dextran sulfate, an experimental AIDS drug that has not been approved for use in the United States. Both dextran sulfate and AL-721 are in demand by AIDS patients, but are not currently being produced by pharmaceutical companies.

228. Anderson, Alun and David Swinbanks. "U.S. Turns Blind Eye to Untested AIDS Treatment Drug Imports." <u>Nature</u>, v. 334, August 4, 1988, p. 369.

The United States government will no longer attempt to halt the import of experimental AIDS drugs that have not been approved by the Food and Drug Administration. The Japanese drug dextran sulfate will now be legally allowed into the country. Some researchers feel that the widespread existence of experimental therapies may harm future drug research.

229. Armstrong, Sue. "Tree Compounds May Strip the Virus of Its Powers." <u>New Scientist</u>, v. 120, November 26, 1988, p. 23.

Three substances derived from plants are showing promise as potential drugs against AIDS. These three compounds are all alkaloids that interfere with the synthesis of sugar chains. They operate against the AIDS virus by inhibiting the enzymes associated with the virus.

230. Barinaga, Marcia. "Placebos Prompt New Protocols for AIDS Drug Tests." Nature, v. 335, October 6, 1988, p. 485.
    People with AIDS often make decisions on whether to comply with the rules of a drug trial based upon their sense of its fairness. This causes problems when using placebos in drug tests because some patients may perform much worse during the trial than others. Self-medication may also lead to problems in determining the true potential of drugs under study.

231. Bartlett, John A. "HIV Therapeutics: An Emerging Science." JAMA: Journal of the American Medical Association, v. 260, November 25, 1988, pp. 3051-3052.
    Since no cure currently exists for AIDS and none is likely to be discovered in the near future, therapies must improve the quality of life for those living with the disease and must also be considered lifelong in duration. The drug zidovudine has been demonstrated to be the most effective so far in meeting these objectives.

232. Booth, William. "An Underground Drug for AIDS." Science, v. 241, September 9, 1988, pp. 1279-1281.
    The Food and Drug Administration has decided to allow AIDS patients to import experimental drugs that have not yet been approved in the United States. The primary drug that will benefit from this program is dextran sulfate, a Japanese product that inhibits the binding of the AIDS virus. This drug will now be available to AIDS patients, even though its effectiveness has yet to be proven.

233. "CD4 Toxin Holds Promise As Treatment for HIV Infection." American Family Physician, v. 38, November 1988, pp. 355-356.
    Using recombinant genetic engineering, researchers have developed a protein that can be used to fight AIDS. It is expected that the CD4 protein will bind to the virus and prevent it from attacking the T-cells.

234. Clark, Matt. "The Drug-Approval Dilemma." Newsweek, v. 112, November 14, 1988, p. 63.
    Pressure is being exerted on the Food and Drug Administration to shorten the time required to approve drugs, especially those for possible use in treating AIDS patients. However, the agency does not want to release any drugs that might later cause harmful side effects. Consumer groups feel that the terminally ill should have the right to try anything to relieve their pain and lengthen their life span.

235. Connor, Steve. "Trial of AIDS Drug Angers Doctors." New Scientist, v. 119, August 25, 1988, p. 22.
    A pharmaceutical company plans to test the experimental AIDS drug dextran sulfate on AIDS patients, but doctors are skeptical of this procedure. They feel that effective clinical trials will be hindered if the drug becomes widely available to potential subjects.

236. Dagani, Ron. "Promising AIDS Drug Begins Human Testing."
<u>Chemical and Engineering News</u>, v. 66, August 15, 1988, p. 6.
   The first human tests of the CD4 protein as a treatment
for AIDS have begun. This protein should bind to the AIDS
virus and prevent it from infecting the T-cells.

237. "Decoy Protein Enters Human Trials." <u>New Scientist</u>, v.
119, August 18, 1988, p. 26.
   Human testing is beginning on the use of the CD4 protein
to stop the reproduction of the AIDS virus. The theory behind
this procedure is that any virus entering the body will bind
to these free proteins and not to the T-cells.

238. "Drug Development Is Too Pro-Business, Consumerists
Assert." <u>Chemical Marketing Reporter</u>, v. 234, November 7,
1988, pp. 7+.
   A new AIDS drug known as CD4-PE has been developed by the
National Institutes of Health.   Critics are afraid that
pharmaceutical companies will charge an outrageous amount of
money for this drug, even though it was created using taxpayer
funding.

239. Ezzell, Carol. "New Clinical Trial Programme for AIDS
in the United States." <u>Nature</u>, v. 336, December 22, 1988, p.
702.
   In an attempt to widen the base of clinical trials of
experimental AIDS drugs, the government has begun a community-
based clinical trial program. Physicians and clinics will
jointly monitor patients who are taking experimental
therapies.

240. Ezzell, Carol. "Tests for New AIDS Treatment Begin in
Three Clinics." <u>Nature</u>, v. 334, August 18, 1988, p. 557.
   Human trials of a new AIDS treatment are beginning. This
treatment uses the CD4 protein of the T-cells. Free proteins
are injected into the bloodstream of infected individuals in
hopes that the virus will bind to these proteins and not to
the T-cells.

241. Ezzell, Carol. "U.S. Looking for Short Cuts to Speed
Drug Approval." <u>Nature</u>, v. 334, August 18, 1988, p. 553.
   The Food and Drug Administration is trying to speed up
approval of drugs used to treat life-threatening illnesses,
including AIDS. This follows the rapid approval of the drug
zidovudine, which was released without completing clinical
trials.

242. "Fansidar-Associated Fatal Reaction in an HIV-Infected
Man." <u>MMWR: Morbidity and Mortality Weekly Report</u>, v. 37,
September 23, 1988, pp. 571-572.
   The drug Fansidar is often used to treat AIDS patients
with pneumocystis carinii pneumonia. A case is presented of
a man who had a fatal allergic reaction to this treatment.

243. "Foreign Drugs Can Enter the U.S." <u>New Scientist</u>, v. 119, August 19, 1988, p. 26.

AIDS patients in the United States may now import drugs from other countries, even if they have not been approved by the Food and Drug Administration. These drugs will be permitted in supplies small enough for one person and cannot be sold to other patients.

244. "French Drug Stunts the Progress of AIDS." <u>New Scientist</u>, v. 119, September 29, 1988, p. 32.

A new drug being tested in France appears to delay the onset of AIDS. Over 40% of the patients using the drug Ditiocarb showed an improved condition after sixteen weeks, as opposed to only 5% of the control group.

245. Gevisser, Mark. "AIDS Movement Seizes Control." <u>Nation</u>, v. 247, December 19, 1988, pp. 677-680.

The Food and Drug Administration has authorized the early release of new experimental drugs to fight AIDS. However, this action will probably not help women and intravenous drug abusers, who have the highest rate of infection. More action is needed to bring treatments to the people most in need of them.

246. Hammer, Joshua. "Inside the Illegal AIDS Drug Trade." <u>Newsweek</u>, v. 112, August 15, 1988, pp. 41-42.

Dextran sulfate is a drug which is thought to inhibit the binding of the AIDS virus. This drug is not approved for use in the United States, but it is being smuggled into the country illegally. The Food and Drug Administration has now approved the import of this drug for personal use by AIDS patients.

247. "Healthy Donors With HIV Help Patients Fight AIDS." <u>New Scientist</u>, v. 120, December 3, 1988, p. 23.

In a limited test, some patients with AIDS have made remarkable recoveries following injections of antibodies from healthy persons infected by the AIDS virus. A larger study of this therapy will begin soon.

248. Hendricks, Melissa. "Two AIDS Drugs May Be Better Than One." <u>Science News</u>, v. 134, September 10, 1988, p. 172.

Although zidovudine prolongs the life of some AIDS patients, it also has several harmful side effects. Some patients who have taken a combination of zidovudine and either dideoxycytidine or amphotericin methyl ester have performed much better than patients taking zidovudine alone. A combination of drugs may be the best treatment for AIDS patients.

249. Hendrickson, Carol. "The AIDS Clinical Trials Unit Experience: Clinical Research and Antiviral Treatment." Nursing Clinics of North America, v. 23, December 1988, pp. 697-706.

As the number of AIDS cases increases, the need for an effective therapy becomes even more apparent. The experiences of a hospital that provided clinical trials of experimental AIDS drugs are presented. Zidovudine is currently the most successful therapy for AIDS patients.

250. "How They Stand: Candidates in the Race to Find a Cure." New Scientist, v. 119, July 7, 1988, p. 33.

Zidovudine, formerly known as AZT, is the most effective drug for treating AIDS patients. The effectiveness of this and several other AIDS drugs are profiled.

251. Joyce, Christopher. "Broader Tests Begin on Antiviral Drug." New Scientist, v. 119, July 21, 1988, p. 36.

The drug dextran sulfate will soon undergo wider testing in patients with AIDS. This drug apparently prevents the AIDS virus from attacking target cells.

252. Kemp, Jim. "The Politics of AIDS Treatment." Christianity and Crisis, v. 48, September 26, 1988, pp. 310-312.

Although the Food and Drug Administration quickly approved the drug zidovudine for AIDS victims, it has moved very slowly on approving other potential treatments. In an effort to make more drugs available, victims will now be able to import drugs from other countries for their personal use against AIDS.

253. Marwick, Charles. "FDA Seeks Swifter Approval of Drugs for Some Life-Threatening or Debilitating Diseases." JAMA: Journal of the American Medical Association, v. 260, November 25, 1988, p. 2976.

The Food and Drug Administration has proposed a method of accelerating drug testing that could cut the time required for approval in half. This will apply only for drugs developed to fight life-threatening diseases such as AIDS.

254. "Pinpointing the Chinks in the Virus's Armor." New Scientist, v. 120, October 8, 1988, p. 24.

The complexity of the AIDS virus and its life cycle may make it vulnerable to some drugs. Several strategies are under investigation, including the destruction of the outer shell of the virus and interfering with the regulatory genes of the virus.

255. Seltzer, Richard. "Government Launches New Steps Against AIDS." <u>Chemical and Engineering News</u>, v. 66, October 31, 1988, p. 16.
   Protests have been held recently in an attempt to receive approval for the release of experimental AIDS drugs. Several government actions have been taken to help speed up the drug evaluation and approval process.

256. Seltzer, Richard. "Protestors Hit FDA for AIDS Drug Policies." <u>Chemical and Engineering News</u>, v. 66, October 17, 1988, p. 5.
   A protest was held at the headquarters of the Food and Drug Administration to rally support for the more rapid approval and release of experimental AIDS drugs and therapies. The government says that it is giving AIDS drugs a high priority, but that it does not want to release potentially dangerous drugs.

257. Shepherd, Frances A. et al. "Combination Chemotherapy and Alpha-Interferon in the Treatment of Kaposi's Sarcoma Associated With Acquired Immune Deficiency Syndrome." <u>Canadian Medical Association Journal</u>, v. 139, October 1, 1988, pp. 635-639.
   Thirteen men with AIDS who exhibited Kaposi's sarcoma were treated with a combination of chemotherapy and alpha-interferon. The median survival time for these patients was 48 weeks. This therapy is not recommended.

258. Spalding, B. J. "The Drug War on AIDS Escalates." <u>Chemical Week</u>, v. 143, September 14, 1988, pp. 14-16.
   Over fifty companies are currently working on a total of 86 potential AIDS drugs and vaccines. Never before has the pharmaceutical industry mobilized so rapidly against a disease. The market for AIDS drugs is expected to grow tremendously.

259. Thompson, Dick. "A Decoy for the Deadly AIDS Virus." <u>Time</u>, v. 132, August 22, 1988, p. 69.
   The CD4 protein can bind to the AIDS virus and stop it from becoming active. A new AIDS therapy is being tested that involves the injection of free CD4 proteins into the bloodstream.

260. United States. Congress. House. Committee on Government Operations. <u>Therapeutic Drugs for AIDS: Development, Testing, and Availability</u>. Washington, D.C.: Government Printing Office, 1988. 448p. Superintendent of Documents number Y4.G74/7:D84/24.
   The complete text of a Congressional hearing on therapies for AIDS patients. The speed of the drug development process must be increased in order to make experimental drugs available to those terminally ill patients who might receive benefits from them.

261. United States. Congress. Senate. Committee on Labor and Human Resources. AIDS Treatment Research and Approval. Washington, D.C.: Government Printing Office, July 13, 1988. 198p. Superintendent of Documents number Y4.L11/4:S.hrg.100-821.
   Potential AIDS drugs need to be made available to those patients who might benefit from their use. The complete text of a Congressional hearing on speeding the availability of AIDS drugs is presented.

262. Vaughan, Christopher. "AIDS Virus Accepts Toxic Trojan Horse." Science News, v. 134, December 3, 1988, p. 358.
   The AIDS virus binds to the CD4 protein of the T-cells, but it has also been shown to bind to free CD4 cells injected into the bloodstream. If a CD4 protein is attached to a toxin, the virus will bind to the protein and the toxin will destroy the virus.

263. Weiss, Rick. "Tailored Toxin Targets HIV-Laden Cells." Science News, v. 134, September 24, 1988, p. 198.
   Through genetic engineering, researchers have created a toxin that targets the surface proteins of the AIDS virus. This toxin may be able to stop infection by the virus.

264. Yarchoan, Robert, Hiroaki Mitsuya, and Samuel Broder. "AIDS Therapies." Scientific American, v. 259, October 1988, pp. 110-119.
   The drug zidovudine is the only therapy that has proven successful in treating AIDS patients. Several potential methods of preventing infection and several other potential AIDS drugs are discussed.

265. Young, Frank E. and S. L. Nightingale. "FDA's Newly Designated Treatment INDs." JAMA: Journal of the American Medical Association, v. 260, July 8, 1988, pp. 224-225.
   Two new experimental drugs have been approved for use with patients facing life-threatening diseases. One of these, trimetrexate glucuromate, appears to be effective for treating AIDS patients suffering from pneumocystis carinii pneumonia.

The Search for an AIDS Vaccine

266. Barnes, Deborah M.   "Another Glitch for AIDS Vaccines?" <u>Science</u>, v. 241, July 29, 1988, pp. 533-534.
   Some AIDS vaccines may actually enhance infection by the virus. Antibodies to the virus have yet to be shown to stop infection. It is not clear how they might aid infection.

267. Coles, Peter. "Paris Retrovirus Conference." <u>Nature</u>, v. 336, November 3, 1988, p. 8.
   Although there is an environment of optimism surrounding AIDS vaccine research, no significant breakthroughs have occurred. Vaccines based on the gp120 protein or on free CD4 proteins have both run into difficulty.

268. "First Trial of Blocking Antibody Dispels Safety Fears." <u>New Scientist</u>, v. 119, July 7, 1988, p. 33.
   The first human tests have been conducted on a new AIDS vaccine. The two patients participating in the test both responded positively. This work could lead to an AIDS vaccine or to a therapy that can be given to those infected by the virus.

269. Kingman, Sharon.   "British Take First Steps Towards a Vaccine." <u>New Scientist</u>, v. 120, October 8, 1988, p. 24.
   Human trials of British AIDS vaccines may begin within the next few years. These vaccines will be based on proteins from the envelope portion of the AIDS virus.

270. Koff, Wayne C. and Daniel F. Hoth.   "Development and Testing of AIDS Vaccines." <u>Science</u>, v. 241, July 22, 1988, pp. 426-432.
   Progress towards an AIDS vaccine has been hindered by a lack of understanding of immunity to the virus, the variations among the different AIDS viruses, and the lack of effective animal models. Vaccine research and testing is reviewed.

271. Matthews, Thomas J. and Dani P. Bolognesi.   "AIDS Vaccines." <u>Scientific American</u>, v. 259, October 1988, pp. 120-127.
   Several potential AIDS vaccines are currently being tested and several others are being studied in the laboratory. Some of the strategies for vaccine development are discussed.

272. Patlak, Margie.   "One Small Step Toward a Vaccine." <u>Discover</u>, v. 9, August 1988, p. 22.
   Daniel Zagury, the researcher who inoculated himself with an experimental AIDS vaccine, has reported that the vaccine has been effective in protecting against infection. The vaccine, which is a genetically engineered cowpox virus, generates a strong immune response.

273. Sarma, Padman, Kenneth J. Cremer, and Jack Gruber.
"Acquired Immunodeficiency Syndrome: Progress and Prospects
for Vaccine Development." Journal of the National Cancer
Institute, **v. 80, October 5, 1988, pp. 1193-1197.**
Several strategies are currently being used in the search
for an AIDS vaccine. An effective animal model is needed to
study the basic mechanisms of the virus and the effectiveness
of various potential vaccines.

274. Zuckerman, Arie J. "Prospects for Vaccines Against HIV."
British Medical Journal, v. 297, July 9, 1988, pp. 86-88.
Several different strategies are being tested in the
search for an AIDS vaccine. Research is continuing using
inactivated live viruses, viruses created through genetic
engineering, hybrid viruses, and novel antigens. Despite this
research, an effective vaccine is not expected to be available
for another ten years.

Origins of the AIDS Virus

275. Essex, Max and Phyllis J. Kanki. "The Origins of the AIDS Virus." <u>Scientific American</u>, v. 259, October 1988, pp. 64-71.

Several viruses similar to the human AIDS virus have been discovered in monkeys. Some of the animal viruses do not cause disease in their hosts. Researchers are searching for other viruses that are similar to the human AIDS virus.

276. Garry, Robert F. et al. "Documentation of an AIDS Virus Infection in the United States in 1968." <u>JAMA: Journal of the American Medical Association</u>, v. 260, October 14, 1988, pp. 2085-2087.

A case has previously been reported of an adolescent male who had died of symptoms similar to AIDS in 1968. Tests of preserved tissues taken from this patient indicate that he had been infected by a virus closely related to the current AIDS virus. It is possible that an immunosuppressive retrovirus existed in the United States before the late 1970s.

277. "Human Viruses Diverged 45 Years Ago." <u>New Scientist</u>, v. 119, July 7, 1988, p. 33.

A computer model has indicated that the HIV-1 and HIV-2 viruses diverged from each other approximately 45 years ago. This date assumes a constant rate of mutation over time.

The HIV-2 and Other AIDS Viruses

278. Connor, Steve. "Britain Puts Off Testing for Second Virus." <u>New Scientist</u>, v. 120, November 26, 1988, p. 22.

The British government has decided that it is unnecessary to test blood for the HIV-2 virus. The costs of such a program would be high and no donated blood has yet tested positive for this virus. Only three cases of AIDS related to HIV-2 have been reported in Britain.

279. Marx, Jean L. "The AIDS Virus Can Take on Many Guises." <u>**Science**</u>**, v. 241, August 26, 1988, pp. 1039-1040.**

The AIDS virus changes its genetic structure frequently, often within a single individual. These variations will hinder efforts to develop an AIDS vaccine and may help to explain some of the pathogenic features of the disease.

280. Marx, Jean L. "Tracking Variation in the AIDS Virus Family." <u>Science</u>, v. 241, August 5, 1988, pp. 659-660.

A possible new AIDS virus has been discovered in West Africa. It is not clear if the new HIV-3 virus causes the disease. In addition, a virus similar to HIV-1 has been isolated that does not appear to be pathogenic.

The Neurological and Psychological Aspects of AIDS

281. "AIDS and the Elusive Power of Belief." <u>Newsweek</u>, v. 112, November 7, 1988, p. 92.

Psychologists have discovered that personality may play a role in survival among AIDS patients. In a study of eighteen men, those with aggressive or narcissistic personalities had higher numbers of certain immune system cells than those patients with other personalities.

282. **Baum, Andrew and Sarah E. A. Nesselhof. "Psychological Research and the Prevention, Etiology, and Treatment of AIDS." <u>American Psychologist</u>, v. 43, November 1988, pp. 900-906.**

Psychological factors are important in all areas of AIDS research, including AIDS prevention, education, and health care. Psychological factors may also play a role in the initial infection and the onset of the disease.

283. Bower, Bruce. "Emotion-Immunity Link in HIV Infection." <u>Science News</u>, v. 134, August 20, 1988, p. 116.

Some of the same psychological factors associated with long-term survival of cancer patients have been linked to long-term survival with AIDS. Anger, vigor, openly displaying emotions, and a denial of the disease have all been linked to a stronger immune system.

284. Brew, Bruce J. et al. "AIDS Dementia Complex." <u>Journal of the Royal College of Physicians</u>, v. 22, July 1988, pp. 140-144.

AIDS dementia complex causes slowed mental capacity, forgetfulness, personality changes, and apathy. This is caused by the direct infection of the brain by the AIDS virus. Although zidovudine has been tested on these patients, no effective therapy has yet been developed.

285. **Catalan, J. "Psychosocial and Neuropsychiatric Aspects of HIV Infection: Review of Their Extent and Implications for Psychiatry." <u>Journal of Psychosomatic Research</u>, v. 32, 1988, pp. 237-248.**

AIDS infection presents a major challenge to health services around the world. It has been known that the virus infects the central nervous system and information is now being gathered on AIDS-related psychiatric disorders. The psychosocial and neurological disorders caused by AIDS are discussed along with their implications for mental health care.

286. Fenton, T. W.   "Psychiatric Aspects of HIV Infection: Implications for the U.K." <u>Journal of the Royal College of Physicians</u>, v. 22, July 1988, pp. 145-148.
     AIDS infection is associated with several psychological reactions, including insecurity, guilt, and helplessness. The virus also causes direct damage to the central nervous system. It seems unlikely that AIDS will place a great burden on psychiatric services in the short term, but the number of cases will certainly rise.

287. Garrett, Jean E. "The AIDS Patient." <u>Nursing 88</u>, v. 18, September 1988, pp. 50-52.
     Nurses must help AIDS patients and their families cope with the psychological stresses caused by the disease. Advice should be nonjudgemental and should be supportive of both the patient and the family.

288. Govoni, Laura A.   "Psychosocial Issues of AIDS in the Nursing Care of Homosexual Men and Their Significant Others." <u>Nursing Clinics of North America</u>, v. 23, December 1988, pp. 749-765.
     The psychological aspects of AIDS present significant problems to caregivers.   Nurses must be aware of the psychological stresses on homosexual men and must apply nursing care within this framework.

289. Grant, Igor et al.   "Human Immunodeficiency Virus-Associated Neurobehavioral Disorder." <u>Journal of the Royal College of Physicians</u>, v. 22, July 1988, pp. 149-157.
     It is clear that the AIDS virus can create primary neurological disorders, but it is unclear how the virus attacks the brain.   Research has shown that neurological problems exist from the earliest stages of infection. It is unclear if zidovudine is effective in treating this aspect of AIDS infection.

290. Green, John and Agnes Kocsis. "Counselling Patients With AIDS-Related Encephalopathy." <u>Journal of the Royal College of Physicians</u>, v. 22, July 1988, pp. 166-168.
     Many patients have a greater fear of AIDS dementia than of death from other secondary infections. Counselling can help patients work through these fears. Patients should be told that the incidence of this syndrome is uncertain, that most people only develop mild symptoms, and that some treatments for AIDS may relieve or reverse this problem.

291. Kiecolt-Glaser, Janice and Ronald Glaser. "Psychological Influences on Immunity." <u>American Psychologist</u>, v. 43, November 1988, pp. 892-898.
     There is solid evidence that psychological factors may influence the immune system. Psychological or behavioral variables may be cofactors of AIDS infection.

292. Mahorney, Steven L. and Jesse O. Cavenar, Jr. "A New and Timely Delusion: The Complaint of Having AIDS." _American Journal of Psychiatry_, v. 145, September 1988, pp. 1130-1132.
Three case of persons who had delusions of AIDS are presented. None of the three were members of high-risk groups and none were actually infected.

293. Martin, John L. "Psychological Consequences of AIDS-Related Bereavement Among Gay Men." _Journal of Consulting and Clinical Psychology_, v. 56, December 1988, pp. 856-862.
In a study of 745 homosexual men in New York City, 27% had experienced the death of a lover or close friend due to AIDS. This caused increased stress and a higher demand for psychological services in this population. It does not appear that homosexual men are adapting psychologically to repeated AIDS-related deaths.

294. Matarazzo, Joseph et al. "APA and AIDS." _American Psychologist_, v. 43, November 1988, pp. 978-982.
The American Psychological Association was one of the first national scientific and professional societies to become involved in the fight against AIDS. The history of that involvement is described.

295. **McArthur, Julie H., John G. Palenicek, and Laura L. Bowersox. "Human Immunodeficiency Virus and the Nervous System."** _**Nursing Clinics of North America**_**, v. 23, December 1988, pp. 823-841.**
The neurological complications of AIDS infection are reviewed. Some of the clinical manifestations of direct infection by the AIDS virus are reported along with possible treatments.

296. McKusick, Leon. "The Impact of AIDS on Practitioner and Client." _American Psychologist_, v. 43, November 1988, pp. 935-940.
AIDS infection can significantly affect the relationship between the patient and the therapist. Knowledge or lack of knowledge about antibody status may lead to anxiety or depression. Therapists must not let their own feelings about AIDS disrupt their professional interactions with their clients.

297. Miller, David ct al. "The Worried Well: Their Identification and Management." _Journal of the Royal College of Physicians_, v. 22, July 1988, pp. 158-165.
Some persons suffer from the delusion that they have AIDS, despite the fact that they show no signs of infection. In most cases, the anxiety about AIDS serves as a channel for guilt about some past behavior.

298. Morgan, Mary K., Michael E. Clark, and Wayne L. Hartman. "AIDS-Related Dementia: A Case Report of Rapid Cognitive Decline." <u>Journal of Clinical Psychology</u>, v. 44, November 1988, pp. 1024-1028.

A case of rapid decline is presented in a patient with AIDS-related dementia. The victim demonstrated a dramatic decline in IQ over a period of six months.

299. Morin, Stephen F. "AIDS: The Challenge to Psychology." <u>American Psychologist</u>, v. 43, November 1988, pp. 838-842.

Psychologists can play a key role in the fight against AIDS. Psychologists can develop programs aimed at changing risky behaviors and can also help develop models of patient care. The greatest challenge will be to alleviate the cultural, social, economic, and political reactions to AIDS.

300. Murphy, Patrice and Kathleen Perry. "Hidden Grievers." <u>Death Studies</u>, v. 12, 1988, pp. 451-462.

Persons who lose a friend or lover from AIDS suffer feelings of loss and grief. A bereavement support group can help survivors recover from the depression of loss due to AIDS.

301. Pearlin, Leonard I., Shirley Semple, and Heather Turner. "Stress and AIDS Caregiving: A Preliminary Overview of the Issues." <u>Death Studies</u>, v. 12, 1988, pp. 501-517.

The loss of a friend or lover from AIDS can create a great deal of stress among the survivors. Specific sources of stress include the demands of caring for the patient, uncertainty over the future, and a disruption of social activities. Support systems are needed for those grieving losses due to AIDS.

302. Pinching, Anthony J. "Neurological Aspects of the Acquired Immune Deficiency Syndrome." <u>Journal of the Royal College of Physicians</u>, v. 22, July 1988, pp. 136-139.

Neurological problems are common among AIDS victims. Patients must be rigorously assessed to determine if infection has occurred and if treatment is required. The options for treating this manifestation of the disease with zidovudine or any other drugs have yet to be established.

303. Pleck, J. H. et al. "AIDS-Phobia, Contact With AIDS, and AIDS-Related Job Stress in Hospital Workers." <u>Journal of Homosexuality</u>, v. 15, 1988, pp. 41-54.

Negative feelings about AIDS and AIDS patients are common among health care workers. This attitude is most common among older staff members who have little contact with AIDS victims. Persons with AIDS-phobia or who have little contact with victims are also more vulnerable to stress.

304. Price, Richard W. and Bruce J. Brew. "The AIDS Dementia Complex." <u>Journal of Infectious Diseases</u>, v. 158, November 1988, pp. 1079-1083.

    To many physicians, the AIDS dementia complex remains ambiguous. It is difficult to diagnose and the treatment for this problem is much less developed than for other manifestations of the disease.

305. Saunders, Judith M. and Stephen L. Buckingham. "When the Depression Turns Deadly." <u>Nursing 88</u>, v. 18, July 1988, pp. 59-64.

    Male AIDS patients have a risk of suicide that is 36 times higher than other men of the same age. Nurses should try to discuss the patient's feelings and should take all talk of suicide seriously. Caregivers cannot restore a long life to their patients, but they can restore a reason for continuing to live.

306. Tross, Susan and Dan A. Hirsch. "Psychological Distress and Neuropsychological Complications of HIV Infection and AIDS." <u>American Psychologist</u>, v. 43, November 1988, pp. 929-934.

    AIDS poses a threat to the psychological health of its victims through discrimination, bereavement, pressure for lifestyle changes, and the progression of the disease itself. Supportive therapy must help victims at all stages of the disease.

Condoms to Prevent the Spread of the AIDS Virus

307. Hacinli, Cynthia. "All Condoms Are Not Alike--Which Test Best?" <u>Mademoiselle</u>, v. 94, November 1988, pp. 133-134.

Condoms prevent the transmission of the AIDS virus, but not all condoms are equally effective. Some tips are offered for selecting and purchasing the safest condoms.

308. Hill, Ronald P. "An Exploration of the Relationship Between AIDS-Related Anxiety and the Evaluation of Condom Advertisements." <u>Journal of Advertising</u>, v. 17, 1988, pp. 35-42.

Advertising for condoms is affected by the level of anxiety about AIDS among consumers. Attitudes toward condom advertising are based on the subject's level of anxiety concerning the spread of AIDS in society, but attitudes about specific brands are related to personal fears of infection.

309. Kalter, Henry D. "Surveillance of Condom Distribution and Usage in Baltimore, Maryland." <u>American Journal of Public Health</u>, v. 78, December 1988, pp. 1596-1597.

A new program has been established to monitor condom distribution and sales. The number of used condoms will also be measured at the city wastewater treatment plant. This will give public health officials an accurate record of actual condom usage.

310. "Media Asked to Promote the Use of Condoms." <u>Editor and Publisher</u>, v. 121, October 8, 1988, p. 16.

The Advertising Council has asked the media to help promote condoms for protection against AIDS. The condom advertising campaign would like to use a combination of television, radio, and print media.

311. "Networks Holding Firm on Condom Advertising." <u>Television/ Radio Age</u>, v. 36, October 17, 1988, p. 40.

Despite changes in advertising regulations, television networks are still not accepting advertisements for condoms. While they do provide public service announcements about AIDS, they feel that condoms are still too controversial.

312. Ngugi, E. N. et al. "Prevention of Transmission of Human Immunodeficiency Virus in Africa: Effectiveness of Condom Promotion and Health Education Among Prostitutes." <u>Lancet</u>, no. 8616, October 15, 1988, pp. 887-890.

Condom usage was measured before and after an AIDS education program aimed at prostitutes was initiated. Condom use was reported to have increased by a factor of three following education efforts. The rate of infection from the virus was found to be much higher in non-condom users.

313. **Valdiserri, Ronald O. et al. "Variables Influencing Condom Use in a Cohort of Gay and Bisexual Men."** <u>American Journal of Public Health</u>, v. 78, July 1988, pp. 801-805.

A survey on safe sex and condom use was conducted among homosexual and bisexual men who practiced anal intercourse. Results were mixed, with 20% of the men reporting constant condom use and up to 50% never using condoms. Condom use is a complex health-related behavior.

AIDS Education Programs

314. Bartnoff, Harvey S. "Health Care Professional Education and AIDS." <u>Death Studies</u>, v. 12, 1988, pp. 547-562.

Health care workers need to learn about AIDS in order to assess the risks of transmission of the virus and to avoid burnout. AIDS education programs are successful in reducing the stresses and fears surrounding the disease.

315. Bock, Barbara and Loren L. Hoch. "Teaching About AIDS." <u>Science and Children</u>, v. 26, September 1988, pp. 22-25.

A sample AIDS education program is presented. Sample materials are provided for discussing AIDS transmission and prevention to various age groups.

316. "California RNs Set the Pace in Education for AIDS." <u>American Journal of Nursing</u>, v. 88, October 1988, pp. 1423+.

Nurses have taken the initiative in educating health care workers about AIDS. A California program uses the train-the-trainer approach to teach others about the disease.

317. "Family Planners Define Their Role in Preventing Viral Spread." <u>New Scientist</u>, v. 119, July 21, 1988, pp. 36-37.

AIDS education programs often fail because their messages do not fit the cultures of those needing the information. Family planning centers, which have already been working with many of the people most in need of such information, might be better able to provide AIDS education to some populations.

318. Flora, June A. and Carl E. Thoresen. "Reducing the Risk of AIDS in Adolescents." <u>American Psychologist</u>, v. 43, November 1988, pp. 965-970.

Preventing the spread of AIDS among adolescents is crucial. Prevention programs must influence diverse populations and must draw from promising programs in other health-related areas, such as those used to teach about smoking and nutrition.

319. "General Statement on Institutional Response to AIDS Revised January 1988." <u>Journal of American College Health</u>, v. 37, November 1988, pp. 121-125.

Institutions of higher education must respond effectively to the threat of AIDS infection. They must institute education programs to teach their community about the disease. They should also provide appropriate medical services for persons who are infected, but they should not use infection status as a criteria for admission.

320. "Halt the AIDS Rampage." School Administrator, v. 45, November 1988, pp. 53-55.

Several guidelines are provided for planning, implementing, and evaluating AIDS education programs. Suggestions are made on appropriate material to be presented to various age groups.

321. Johnson, Jeffrey A. et al. "A Program Using Medical Students to Teach High School Students About AIDS." Journal of Medical Education, v. 63, July 1988, pp. 522-530.

Describes a pilot project in which twenty medical school students taught AIDS prevention measures to high school students. The high school students were interested in AIDS and liked having medical school students as teachers.

322. Kerr, Diane L. "Summary of ASHA Members' Results on the ASHA AIDS Education Needs Assessment." Journal of School Health, v. 58, October 1988, p. 315.

A survey of members of the American School Health Association reveals that 62% desired information on how to plan an AIDS education program. AIDS policy statements and training were also desired by the majority of respondents.

323. Lohrmann, David K. "AIDS Education at the Local Level: The Pragmatic Issues." Journal of School Health, v. 58, October 1988, pp. 330-334.

In order to establish an AIDS program at the local level, several issues must be resolved. The school needs to establish an AIDS policy, it must discuss morality, values, and ethics, and it must relate AIDS instruction to other health instruction.

324. Matheny, Samuel C. and Nancy S. Kilpatrick. "HRSA AIDS Curriculum Conferences Assist Primary Care Health Professionals." Public Health Reports, v. 103, September/October 1988, pp. 553-556.

Public health professionals have been thrust into the center of the fight against AIDS. They must know how to protect themselves, how to diagnose and treat infected persons, prevention methods for families and friends of the infected, and how to counsel those who have been infected but who do not have the disease. The federal government has established an AIDS education curriculum to teach these concepts to health care workers.

325. "Public Knowledge About AIDS Improving: AMA Survey." American Pharmacy, v. 28, October 1988, p. 50.

Over 80% of adults surveyed indicated that they knew something about AIDS. This represents a 10% increase from the responses made during the previous year. This rise indicates that AIDS education programs are achieving their goals.

326. Rienzo, Barbara A. and Steve M. Dorman. "Ten Consequences of the AIDS Crisis for the Health Education Profession." Journal of School Health, v. 58, October 1988, pp. 335-338.
   AIDS has changed the role of the health education professional. It requires the development of new media for educating about health, an increased emphasis on accurate and timely information, and a new look at moral and ethical issues.

327. Schietinger, Helen et al. "A Strategy for Educating Health Care Providers About AIDS: The California Nurses Association's AIDS Train the Trainer Program." Nursing Clinics of North America, v. 23, December 1988, pp. 779-787.
   The California Nurses Association has developed an effective AIDS education program aimed at health care providers. Each person who takes the course becomes an instructor who teaches others. This method spreads the information quickly and cost-effectively.

328. Shayne, Vivian T. and Barbara J. Kaplan. "AIDS Education for Adolescents." Youth and Society, v. 20, December 1988, pp. 180-208.
   Adolescents are at risk for infection by the AIDS virus, but most do not feel that the disease will directly affect them. Educational programs aimed at changing adolescent behaviors are needed in the schools, in community organizations, and in the media.

329. Smithson, R. D. "Public and Health Staff Knowledge About AIDS." Community Medicine, v. 10, August 1988, pp. 221-227.
   The general public's knowledge level about AIDS is fairly high. The methods of transmission of the virus appear to be well known, although many people still believe that the virus may be transmitted by donating blood. Education programs must now concentrate on changing the behaviors that place the patient at risk for AIDS.

330. United States. Office of Technology Assessment. How Effective Is AIDS Education? Washington, D.C.: Government Printing Office, May 1988. 128p. Superintendent of Document number Y3.T22/2:2Ac7/3.
   AIDS education programs have led to a significant increase in the knowledge of the public about the disease. However, some misconceptions about the methods of transmission still exist. Only a minority of the public has changed its behavior to avoid becoming infected.

331. Vener, Arthur and Krupka, Lawrence. "AIDS Knowledge." <u>American Biology Teacher</u>, v. 50, October 1988, pp. 426-431.
    An AIDS knowledge test was given to over 1,000 college students. On the average, 71% of the questions were answered correctly. Biology teachers must work to increase knowledge levels even further.

332. White, David M. et al. "AIDS and the Immune System." <u>Journal of School Health</u>, v. 58, October 1988, pp. 339-340.
    Explaining the complicated nature of the immune system is quite difficult. A model of the immune system as a battleground is proposed to better help students understand how the AIDS virus infects the body.

333. Windom, Robert E. "A Call to Arms for Health Care Workers." <u>Public Health Reports</u>, v. 103, July/August 1988, p. 337.
    Health care professionals form the front lines in the war against AIDS. They must make sure that all of the public is accurately informed about the disease and should actively participate in community education programs.

AIDS and the Schools

334. "Acquired Immunodeficiency Syndrome Education in Schools." Pediatrics, v. 82, August 1988, pp. 278-280.
    The schools should make AIDS education programs part of their total health education plan. Some specific guidelines are presented on the training of health care workers and teachers and on integrating AIDS education into the curriculum. These programs should be evaluated on a periodic basis and should be constantly updated to conform with current knowledge about the disease.

335. Adams, Richard, Marilyn Marcontel, and Alfreda L. Price. "The Impact of AIDS on School Health Services." Journal of School Health, v. 58, October 1988, pp. 341-343.
    Changing behavior through education is the only hope of stopping the spread of AIDS. School health personnel can have a dramatic effect on preventing AIDS among adolescents.

336. Bennett, Joseph L. "The Best Defense." Currents, v. 14, July/August 1988, pp. 48-50.
    Many schools have begun AIDS education programs to help stop the spread of the disease. Public relations directors must work with educators to promote health education and AIDS prevention.

337. Black, Jeffrey L. and Lorraine H. Jones. "HIV Infection: Educational Programs and Policies for School Personnel." Journal of School Health, v. 58, October 1988, pp. 317-322.
    Schools are at the front lines of defense against the spread of AIDS. School staff need to be kept current on the disease and must transmit information about the methods of transmission to their students.

338. Brown, Larry K. and Gregory K. Fritz. "AIDS Education in the Schools." Clinical Pediatrics, v. 27, July 1988, pp. 311-316.
    Pediatricians will become more involved with schools as they become more involved in AIDS education. This literature review covers material on student knowledge levels, education programs, and drug abuse prevention.

339. Carter, Linda K. "A Case of AIDS." Currents, v. 14, July/August 1988, pp. 42-46.
    Several institutions have adopted the AIDS guidelines established by the American Council on Education and the American College Health Association. A campus response to AIDS must include the formation of a campus AIDS committee, the development of an AIDS education program, and the creation of a flexible AIDS policy.

340. Essex, Nathan L. "Students With AIDS: An Administrative Dilemma." <u>Principal</u>, v. 68, September 1988, pp. 14-15.
    The presence of students with AIDS in the public schools has created problems for teachers, parents, and other students. School administrators must provide an adequate education to students with AIDS, but must also protect other children from infection. Guidelines are provided for developing an AIDS policy.

341. Futrell, Mary H. "AIDS Education Through Schools." <u>Journal of School Health</u>, v. 58, October 1988, pp. 324-326.
    AIDS education programs must motivate students to avoid risky behaviors. Schools, parents, and the community must all become involved if the program is to be successful.

342. "HIV-Related Beliefs, Knowledge, and Behaviors Among High School Students." <u>MMWR: Morbidity and Mortality Weekly Report</u>, v. 37, December 2, 1988, pp. 717-721.
    A survey was conducted to determine student knowledge levels regarding AIDS. Most knew that AIDS is transmitted by sexual intercourse or through needle sharing, but less than one-half knew that the virus could not be transmitted through insect bites, donating blood, or using public toilets.

343. "Instruction About AIDS Within the School Curriculum." <u>Journal of School Health</u>, v. 58, October 1988, p. 323.
    The primary source of information on AIDS for children must be parents and other caregivers. Schools should provide accurate information about AIDS within the curriculum, but the decision on what is to be included should be made on an individual basis by each school district.

344. Katzman, Elaine M., Marion Mulholland, and Edward M. Sutherland. "College Students and AIDS: A Preliminary Survey of Knowledge, Attitudes, and Behavior." <u>Journal of American College Health</u>, v. 37, November 1988, pp. 127-130.
    A telephone survey was conducted to determine the knowledge level that college students have about AIDS. Nearly 90% of those surveyed could identify the routes of transmission of the virus and almost all knew that condoms protected against infection. They also expressed a strong concern over the spread of the virus among their peers.

345. Leslie, Connie. "Amid the Ivy, Cases of AIDS." <u>Newsweek</u>, v. 112, November 14, 1988, p. 65.
    College students are at a high risk for AIDS, with approximately one of every 300 students already infected. Despite the risk of AIDS, one-half of the nation's colleges do not yet offer any AIDS information programs.

346. Phelps, Mary-Ellen. "The Little Town That Could." <u>Christianity and Crisis</u>, v. 48, July 4, 1988, pp. 230-231.
　　　　A small town in Maryland reacted well to a case of a child with AIDS in its schools. Community members were concerned, but they did not try to keep the child out of the classroom.

347. "A Scary Little Survey of AIDS on Campus." <u>U.S. News and World Report</u>, v. 105, November 14, 1988, p. 12.
　　　　Preliminary results from a survey of students on college campuses indicate that three of every 1,000 students have been infected by the AIDS virus. The sexual activity of college students puts this population at a high risk for infection.

348. Strope, John L. Jr. "Teachers With AIDS." <u>West's Education Law Reporter</u>, v. 47, 1988, pp. 827-835.
　　　　Teachers with AIDS are protected under section 504 of the Rehabilitation Act of 1973. Teachers cannot be isolated, transferred, suspended, or terminated because they have AIDS. Schools are bound by the same regulations and must treat their employees in the same manner as any other employer.

AIDS in the Workplace

349. "AIDS in the Workplace: Guidelines." Journal of
Occupational Medicine, v. 30, July 1988, pp. 578-579.
     General guidelines are provided to help companies
establish AIDS policies. Employee education is emphasized and
mandatory testing is not recommended. Safety measures should
be taken to prevent occupational transmission of the virus and
the immune status of all employees should remain confidential.

350. Backer, Thomas E. "Managing AIDS at Work." American
Psychologist, v. 43, November 1988, pp. 983-987.
     Many employers are developing AIDS policies and programs.
Challenges to effective programs include the stigma of the
disease, financial considerations, and legal liabilities.
Strategic planning is helpful for employers dealing with AIDS.

351. Bantsari, Lee A. "AIDS in the Workplace: Education Eases
Fear." Pulp and Paper, v. 62, August 1988, p. 7.
     AIDS has reached the American workplace. It is a social
issue that requires education of both management and
employees. Companies and unions need to develop AIDS policies
and carry on an active dialogue about the disease.

352. "Battling AIDS Into the Next Century." Risk Management,
v. 35, December 1988, pp. 56-58.
     By 1992, over 365,000 cases of AIDS will have been
reported in the United States and 263,000 people will have
died from the disease. It is important for employers to
protect themselves against the high cost of AIDS insurance
claims. It is also important to develop an AIDS policy that
informs employees about the real risks of the disease.

353. Brockhoeft, John E. "AIDS in the Workplace: Legal
Limitations on Employer Actions." American Business Law
Journal, v. 26, Summer 1988, pp. 255-303.
     Employers who fire, transfer, or place AIDS patients on
indefinite sick leave are liable for legal action from the
employee. Employees with AIDS are protected under federal
legislation that protects the handicapped. An employer must
have a legitimate cause for action to terminate or remove an
employee with AIDS.

354. Chenoweth, David. "AIDS Brings New Conflicts, Employer
Responsibilities Into Nation's Workplace." Occupational
Health and Safety, v. 57, July 1988, p. 34.
     Employers must protect the rights of their employees and
work within the context of the law. Mandatory AIDS testing
is not recommended, even though insurance rates will rise due
to the high costs of AIDS. Education is the best method for
reducing the number of AIDS cases among employees.

355. Ferrill, Harve A. "Corporate Myopia Is Not the Answer." <u>Management Review</u>, v. 77, December 1988, pp. 54-55.

AIDS will soon become a problem for all corporations. AIDS costs are rising and insurers are restricting coverage of the disease. Home care should be encouraged and employees should pressure insurers into covering this type of care.

356. Friddle, Jamie et al. "How Companies Can Ease the Burden of AIDS at Work." <u>Occupational Health and Safety</u>, v. 57, July 1988, pp. 12-19+.

The problem of employees who have AIDS or who have become infected by the AIDS virus has raised questions for many companies. Employees are protected under federal legislation and must be treated like any other handicapped workers. All employees need to be educated about the disease.

357. Holtom, Robert B. "AIDS in the Workplace." <u>Best's Review (Property/Casualty Insurance Edition)</u>, v. 89, September 1988, pp. 96-100.

To date, very few companies have formulated AIDS policies. Companies must ensure that their employees learn the facts about AIDS in order to protect themselves from legal action related to the disease.

358. Marinelli, L. et al. "Transmission of AIDS in the Aviation Environment." <u>Aviation, Space, and Environmental Medicine</u>, v. 59, July 1988, pp. 683-684.

AIDS is transmitted through sexual contact, contaminated blood, and from mother to child during pregnancy. The virus is not transmitted during the casual workplace environment. Aviation industry employees who have AIDS are not a threat to coworkers.

359. Miller, William H. "Facing Up to AIDS." <u>Industry Week</u>, v. 237, September 19, 1988, pp. 19-20.

Although many large companies have begun to implement AIDS education and prevention programs, few firms have adopted a written AIDS policy. Several steps for developing an AIDS policy are presented.

360. Minetos, Peter. "Corporate America vs. AIDS." <u>Safety and Health</u>, v. 138, December 1988, pp. 34-36.

Corporations can take a leadership role in the fight against AIDS. Companies must protect the rights of their employees and must also educate the workforce about the disease. Testing should be voluntary and all results should be confidential.

361. Morgan, David R. and John Dawson. "Occupational Health Aspects of the Human Immunodeficiency Virus and AIDS." Annals of Occupational Hygiene, **v. 32, 1988, pp. 69-82.**

AIDS is spread through sexual intercourse, infected blood or blood products, and from mother to child at or before birth. There is also evidence that the virus may be transmitted to persons in certain occupations, such as the health care profession. Occupational safety professionals have a key role to play in preventing the occupational spread of the disease.

362. Patterson, Bill. "AIDS in the Workplace: Is Your Company Prepared to Handle the World's Greatest Health Threat?" Professional Safety, **v. 33, October 1988, p. 33.**

Only 10% of all corporations in the United States have developed an AIDS plan. Employees must be aware of the facts about AIDS if the company is to avoid lawsuits. An AIDS policy written before a case appears is as good as insurance against the disease.

363. Redeker, James R. and Jonathan A. Segal. "The Legal Ramifications of AIDS Discrimination." Business and Society Review, **v. 65, Spring 1988, pp. 18-24.**

Employers should develop AIDS policies before they have any employees who contract the disease. Employees with AIDS are protected under federal legislation protecting the handicapped. Testing is not permitted unless it is for a specific job-related purpose. Education and safety programs can help employers deal with AIDS.

364. Shalowitz, Deborah. "NAM Urges Corporate AIDS Strategies." Business Insurance, **v. 22, September 26, 1988, p. 22.**

Companies should develop AIDS policies even if they have no employees who are currently infected. This provides legal protection for both the company and the employee. An educational program is an essential component of any corporate AIDS policy.

365. Stevens, George E. "Understanding AIDS." Personnel Administrator, **v. 33, August 1988, pp. 84-88.**

Companies must be aware of the legal implications of employees with AIDS. AIDS victims are protected under laws dealing with the rights of the handicapped. This is complicated by a Department of Justice ruling that states that the ability to transmit a virus is not protected. Employers should learn the facts about the disease and should protect the confidentiality of their employees.

366. Wagel, William H.   "AIDS: Setting Policy, Educating Employees at Bank of America." <u>Personnel</u>, v. 65, August 1988, pp. 4-8.

   The Bank of America has set the pace for the corporate response to the AIDS epidemic. The personnel policies and education programs developed by this company are profiled.

Health Care Workers and AIDS

367. Auman, Jane. "Health Care Workers and AIDS." <u>Business Insurance</u>, v. 22, September 26, 1988, p. 28.

Despite the low incidence of occupational exposure to the AIDS virus for health care workers, there is still a real danger of infection. Hospitals should initiate AIDS policies and should follow the safety guidelines established by the Centers for Disease Control.

368. Barnes, Deborah M. "Health Workers and AIDS: Questions Persist." <u>Science</u>, v. 241, July 8, 1988, pp. 161-162.

A laboratory worker at the National Institutes of Health has become infected with the AIDS virus through occupational exposure. Of over 2,200 people who have been injured while working with infected products, only sixteen have become infected. It is not clear why some workers become infected and others do not.

369. Bolle, Jacques L. "Supporting the Deliverers of Care: Strategies to Support Nurses and Prevent Burnout." <u>Nursing Clinics of North America</u>, v. 23, December 1988, pp. 843-850.

Nurses who treat AIDS victims are subject to stress and burnout. Sources and methods of preventing burnout are presented. Caregivers must support each other in order to avoid being overwhelmed by the stresses caused by the disease.

370. Clever, Linda H. "AIDS: A Special Challenge for Health Care Workers." <u>Death Studies</u>, v. 12, 1988, pp. 519-529.

Health care workers are at risk for AIDS through occupational exposure as well as through their own individual lifestyles. Recommendations are made for health care workers to avoid infection and maintain an ethical and professional relationship with AIDS patients.

371. Gerbert, Barbara et al. "Why Fear Persists: Health Care Professionals and AIDS." <u>JAMA: Journal of the American Medical Association</u>, v. 260, December 16, 1988, pp. 3481-3483.

Some health care workers have refused to carry out their responsibilities due to a fear of AIDS. This fear is promoted by the fact that health care authorities downplay the real risk of exposure, that infection control procedures do not guarantee against transmission, and that communication between authorities and health care workers is hindered by the differing goals of the two groups.

372. Green, Margaret A. and Thomas G. Robins. "Recommendations for Prevention of HIV Transmission in Health Care Settings." _Journal of Occupational Medicine_, v. 30, July 1988, pp. 587-588.

Health care workers are protected under the federal "right to know" laws and should be aware of any patients infected by the AIDS virus. Warning labels should be placed on all bodily fluids taken from AIDS patients in order to alert health care personnel of the possible dangers of infection.

373. "Guidelines to Prevent Simian Immunodeficiency Virus Infection in Laboratory Workers and Animal Handlers." _MMWR: Morbidity and Mortality Weekly Report_, v. 37, November 18, 1988, pp. 693-694+.

The expanding use of the Simian AIDS virus as a model for human AIDS has raised concerns about possible human infections by this virus. Although no case of a human infected by the animal virus has been reported, safety recommendations are made to protect laboratory workers.

374. Henderson, Deborah J. "HIV Infection: Risks to Health Care Workers and Infection Control." _Nursing Clinics of North America_, v. 23, December 1988, pp. 767-777.

Although the risk of transmission of the AIDS virus in the health care environment is very small, the risk does exist. Safety precautions are recommended to minimize the chance of infection.

375. "HIV Transmission in Hospitals: African Study Shows Reassuring Results." _New Scientist_, v. 120, November 26, 1988, p. 23.

Over 8% of a group of 2,000 African hospital workers were infected by the AIDS virus at the end of 1986. This figure reflects the infection rate of the total population and does not imply a high risk of occupational exposure.

376. Katzin, Louise. "HIV Risk (Still) Low for Health Care Workers." _American Journal of Nursing_, v. 88, July 1988, p. 950.

The rate of occupational transmission of the AIDS virus to health care workers is very low. Only four of 1,070 persons who were at risk for infection have tested positive.

377. Loewy, Erich H. "Risk and Obligation: Health Professionals and the Risk of AIDS." _Death Studies_, v. 12, 1988, pp. 531-545.

Health care workers have historically treated patients when a reasonable risk of infection has been present. This attitude should not be changed with respect to AIDS. The health care community's views towards justice and professionalism will define its response to AIDS.

378. Marcus, Ruthanne. "Surveillance of Health Care Workers Exposed to Blood From Patients Infected With the Human Immunodeficiency Virus." New England Journal of Medicine, v. 319, October 27, 1988, pp. 1118-1123.

In a study of 1,201 health care workers who had been exposed to blood or other bodily fluids taken from AIDS patients, only 0.4% had become infected. Risk of infection is real but very low and may be minimized by following infection control procedures.

379. Miles, Steven H. "The Medical Profession's Duty to HIV-Infected Persons." Journal of Medical Education, v. 63, July 1988, p. 573.

AIDS creates an ethical problem for physicians, who must weigh the risk of occupational exposure against the professional mission of treating the ill. This duty of treatment must be taught to all future generations of health care workers.

380. N'Galy, Bosenge et al. "Human Immunodeficiency Virus Infection Among Employees in an African Hospital." New England Journal of Medicine, v. 319, October 27, 1988, pp. 1123-1127.

Over 2,000 health care employees at a Kinshasa hospital were tested for infection by the AIDS virus. Between 1984 and 1986, infection rates increased from 6.4% to 8.7%. This is equivalent to the infection rate in the population as a whole and is not due to occupational exposure.

381. "Pediatric Guidelines for Infection Control of Human Immunodeficiency Virus (Acquired Immunodeficiency Virus) in Hospitals, Medical Offices, Schools, and Other Settings." Pediatrics, v. 82, November 1988, pp. 801-807.

AIDS has been diagnosed in over 900 children under thirteen years of age in the United States. The risk of infection to health care workers from these children is very low, but some precautions should still be followed. Specific guidelines are presented for health care workers in various treatment situations.

382. "Professional Responsibility in Treating AIDS Patients." Journal of Medical Education, v. 63 July 1988, pp. 587-590.

Health care personnel and students have a responsibility to provide care to all patients regardless of their diagnosis. Medical schools must ensure that all students understand this basic principle. They must also teach the students about the realities of the occupational risk of contracting AIDS.

383. Ratzan, Richard M. and Henry Schneiderman. "AIDS, Autopsies, and Abandonment." <u>JAMA: Journal of the American Medical Association</u>, v. 260, December 16, 1988, pp. 3466-3469.

Although doctors are at a very low risk for AIDS, a great deal of fear exists within the profession. Physicians have an ethical responsibility to treat and care for all patients, even when their diseases pose a personal risk to the physician.

384. Shulman, Lawrence C. and Joanne E. Mantell. "The AIDS Crisis: A United States Health Care Perspective." <u>Social Sciences and Medicine</u>, v. 26, 1988, pp. 979-988.

AIDS has taken its toll on the health care profession in terms of stress, anxiety, and workload. Hospitals have had to assume the major responsibility for AIDS care, straining their already slim resources. The health care system is being slowly restructured to provide more community-based alternative care facilities.

385. "Updated Guidelines to Prevent AIDS in Health Care Settings." <u>American Family Physician</u>, v. 38, September 1988, pp. 377-378.

The Centers for Disease Control has revised its safety guidelines to protect health care workers from infection by the AIDS virus. Blood and other bodily fluids need to be handled carefully, protective barriers should be used to reduce exposure, and gloves should be used during all phlebotomies.

386. Young, G. Stewart, Carla R. Mond, and Arthur D. Schwope. "Personal Protection Is a Vital Issue in the Fight Against Infection." <u>Occupational Health and Safety</u>, v. 57, August 1988, pp. 38-43.

Concerns over the possible infection of health care workers by the AIDS virus have led to an increased emphasis on safety precautions to protect from infection. The guidelines created by the Centers for Disease Control are discussed along with the safety features of various types of rubber gloves.

AIDS in Prisons

387. Baker, Charles J. and Barry Nidorf. "AIDS Policies for Juveniles: L.A. County Examines the Issues." <u>Corrections Today</u>, v. 50, August 1988, pp. 190-196.

Mass screening and testing of juveniles in detention facilities is not warranted. The confidentiality of anyone infected by the AIDS virus must be protected. Inmates who test positive do not need to be isolated from the rest of the population.

388. Coughlin, Thomas A., III. "AIDS in Prisons: One Correctional Administrator's Recommended Policies and Procedures." <u>Judicature</u>, v. 72, June/July 1988, pp. 63-66+.

The New York State prison system currently has over 500 inmates with AIDS. Inmates who are physically fit are kept in the general prison population. Mass testing of inmates is not justified.

389. Hornblum, Allen M. "Philadelphia's AIDS Policy: A Goode Decision?" <u>Corrections Today</u>, v. 50, December 1988, pp. 88-90.

Philadelphia prison authorities have decided to distribute condoms and needle sterilization kits to inmates in their efforts to stop the spread of AIDS. Some prison officials in other jurisdictions feel that this sends a message to prisoners that homosexuality and drug abuse will be tolerated.

390. Milne, Kirsty. "Life Sentence: Prisoners With AIDS." <u>New Statesman and Society</u>, v. 1, October 7, 1988, pp. 22-23.

The British prison system isolates prisoners with AIDS from the rest of the prison population. New prisoners who are members of high risk groups are required to take an AIDS blood test. Prisoners who become seriously ill are transferred to a hospital.

The Ethical, Social, and Religious Aspects of AIDS

391. Annas, George J. "AIDS, Judges, and the Right to Medical Care." Hastings Center Report, v. 18, August/September 1988, pp. 20-22.

There is no right to medical care written into the Constitution, even in emergency cases. Waiting lists for beds in AIDS clinics are acceptable as long as the decisions on who will be accepted are carried out consistently. Hospitals are also not legally required to make experimental drugs available to dying patients.

392. Annas, George J. "Not Saints, But Healers: The Legal Duties of Health Care Professionals in the AIDS Epidemic." American Journal of Public Health, v. 78, July 1988, pp. 844-849.

Health professionals have the right to treat or not to treat patients based on mutual consent. The only exception to this rule is in the emergency room, where all patients have a legal right to treatment. However, medical ethics policies written by professional associations tend to require treatment of all patients.

393. Fehren, Henry. "Aids for AIDS." U.S. Catholic, v. 53, August 1988, pp. 40-42.

The church should not condemn homosexuals and AIDS patients, but should treat them as Christ would have treated them. All of the sick should receive care and compassion, not just those who agree with specific church doctrines.

394. Fineberg, Harvey V. "The Social Dimensions of AIDS." Scientific American, v. 259, October 1988, pp. 128-134.

The AIDS crisis identifies weaknesses and biases in our social system. Education programs are the best weapons against AIDS, but the issues of drug abuse and homosexuality are offensive to some people. The rights of AIDS patients must always be protected.

395. Giese, William. "AIDS and Home Buyers." Changing Times, v. 42, October 1988, p. 18.

Some real estate agents are being pressured to disclose whether a home has previously been occupied by an AIDS victim. There is no evidence for transmission of the virus through casual contact, but many buyers are afraid to purchase a home formerly belonging to someone with AIDS.

396. Hancock, Lee. "Incarnate Suffering and Faith." Christianity and Crisis, v. 48, July 4, 1988, pp. 240-242.

The church has been conspicuously absent from the war on AIDS. The church must not view AIDS as God's punishment for sin, but as a disease that afflicts mankind and whose victims must be healed.

397. Howell, Joel D. and Carl Cohen. "What Is the Difference Between an HIV and a CBC?" Hastings Center Report, v. 18, August/September 1988, pp. 18-20.

Hospitalized patients should give their consent before being tested for infection by the AIDS virus. Consent is required because this procedure places the patient at greater risk than routine blood testing. Patients should be informed of their infection status when it is known.

398. James, Ann M. "AIDS Raises Policy Issues for Many Hospital Departments." Healthcare Financial Management, v. 42, November 1988, pp. 60-64.

AIDS presents several ethical problems for health care administrators. The questions of whether to inform patients of infection, to test for infection, to protect employees, and to protect the privacy of the patient are all discussed.

399. Keller, M. Jean. "The Psychosocial Implications of AIDS on Leisure Services." Parks and Recreation, v. 23, December 1988, pp. 36-39.

AIDS poses a threat to the provision of recreation services. Both leaders and participants must be aware of the facts of the disease. Precautions should be taken to prevent transmission of the virus, but persons with AIDS should not be excluded from leisure activities.

400. Kenkelen, Bill. "Dilemma for Religious Orders: To Test Or Not to Test for AIDS." National Catholic Reporter, v. 24, pp. 1+.

Some male religious orders are beginning to test applicants for exposure to the AIDS virus. Many are testing to avoid the trauma and expense of having members with AIDS. The Catholic Church has gone on record as opposing mandatory AIDS testing.

401. Loewy, Erich H. "AIDS and the Human Community." Social Sciences and Medicine, v. 27, 1988, pp. 297-303.

The ethical response of a community to the AIDS epidemic is related to the structure of the community and its notions of justice. Communities which hold freedom to be an absolute will avoid mandatory AIDS testing, whereas those that feel threatened by the disease will resort to extreme measures to control infection.

402. Melton, Gary B. "Ethical and Legal Issues in AIDS-Related Practice." American Psychologist, v. 43, November 1988, pp. 941-947.

Psychologists should strive to protect the privacy of their clients and promote the general welfare of patients with AIDS. If a breach of confidence is required, it should be no greater than necessary. Psychologists should become trained in the delivery of AIDS-related services.

403. Miramontes, Helen. "Needed: Effective National Policy on AIDS/HIV Infection." <u>Nursing Outlook</u>, v. 36, November/December 1988, pp. 262-263+.

AIDS is not only the most important medical problem of our time, it is also a great social issue. Some of the ethical issues raised by AIDS testing, education, and funding are discussed.

404. Moriarty, Mary-Beth. "Why AIDS Wracks the Conscience of Nursing." <u>RN</u>, v. 51, October 1988, pp. 58-65.

AIDS is treated differently than other diseases because it is linked to socially unacceptable sexual and drug use behaviors. Nurses must provide treatment to patients but must also protect themselves from infection. As the number of AIDS cases increases, the number of nurses who will be facing personal ethical questions will also increase.

405. Muck, Terry. "AIDS: Evangelical Attitudes." <u>Christianity Today</u>, v. 32, November 18, 1988, p. 15.

A survey of evangelical christians indicated that the majority were aware of the basic facts about AIDS. They felt that the Church should show compassion to victims and should promote fidelity and abstinence. Over one-third of the respondents believed that AIDS is a judgement from God for past sins.

406. **Murphy, Timothy F. "Is AIDS a Just Punishment?" <u>Journal of Medical Ethics</u>, v. 14, September 1988, pp. 154-160.**

Some religious and philosophical arguments view AIDS as a punishment from God for immoral behaviors. These theories are not complete and do not stand up to careful scrutiny. From a logical and philosophical perspective, these arguments cannot be accurate.

407. Northrop, Cynthia E. "Rights Versus Regulation: Confidentiality in the Age of AIDS." <u>Nursing Outlook</u>, v. 36, July/August 1988, p. 208.

Nurses must observe confidentiality when working with AIDS patients. The case of a nurse who informed a hospital that a prospective employee was infected is discussed. This action resulted in a lawsuit against the hospital.

408. **Reisman, Elizabeth C. "Ethical Issues Confronting Nurses." <u>Nursing Clinics of North America</u>, v. 23, December 1988, pp. 789-802.**

Nurses are morally obligated to provide care for AIDS patients, even when care of the patient involves a personal risk to themselves. Nurses must also respect the patient's rights of confidentiality and privacy.

409. Schietinger, Helen. "Housing for People With AIDS." <u>Death Studies</u>, v. 12, 1988, pp. 481-499.

Many AIDS victims become homeless through financial losses and discrimination. The Shanti project in San Francisco was begun to care for homeless AIDS victims. This program is profiled as a model for other AIDS housing programs.

410. Sontag, Susan. "AIDS and Its Metaphors." <u>New York Review of Books</u>, **v. 35, October 27, 1988, pp. 89-99.**

AIDS is commonly understood as a modern plague. This concept of AIDS has an underlying moral theme dealing with its sexual transmission. Epidemics such as AIDS often cause fear and intolerance among those who are not infected.

411. Swing, William E. "Silence in the Sanctuaries." <u>Christianity and Crisis</u>, **v. 48, July 4, 1988, pp. 225-227.**

The church has done little about AIDS because it is afraid to venture into issues dealing with human sexuality. While all other sectors of society discuss the disease, the church remains silent. The church needs to act before AIDS moves beyond homosexuals and drug abusers.

412. Wiley, Katherine et al. "Care of AIDS Patients: Student Attitudes." <u>Nursing Outlook</u>, v. 36, September/October 1988, pp. 244-245.

In a survey of nursing students, over one-half of the respondents felt that health care workers should be able to refuse treatment to AIDS patients. Nursing faculty must reinforce the ethical and moral issues involved in providing health care.

The Political and Legal Aspects of AIDS

413. "AIDS's Rights--And Ours." <u>National Review</u>, v. 40, November 7, 1988, p. 18.

A proposition on the California ballot would require the reporting of all AIDS patients if passed. Some feel that this law would drive AIDS underground, but passage would require those testing positive to become informed of their condition.

414. Allen, Glen. "AIDS and Civil Rights." <u>Maclean's</u>, v. 101, October 3, 1988, p. 50.

Health authorities in Canada have notified police of a man who continued to engage in sexual activity with several women even after he knew that he was infected by the AIDS virus. In this case, public health was ruled to be more important than patient confidentiality.

415. Anderson, Alun. "Congress Passes Bill to Fight AIDS." <u>Nature</u>, v. 335, October 20, 1988, p. 657.

A comprehensive AIDS bill has passed Congress, but some controversial sections have had to be removed as a compromise with conservative members. The final bill will increase the number of AIDS research personnel and will provide additional research funds.

416. Anderson, Alun and Marcia Barinaga. "AIDS Bill Wins Overwhelming Congressional Support." <u>Nature</u>, v. 335, September 29, 1988, p. 386.

For the first time, an AIDS bill has passed both the House and Senate by a wide majority. The bill calls for the hiring of more AIDS researchers, faster approval of new drugs, and the testing of persons who have a high risk of exposure to the virus.

417. Beardsley, Tim. "AIDS and the Election: Currently Neglected." <u>Scientific American</u>, v. 259, October 1988, pp. 14+.

Neither presidential candidate has paid much attention to AIDS, despite the fact that over 250,000 people are expected to die of the disease during the next four years. Both candidates have endorsed the recommendations of the Presidential Commission on AIDS, but the Democrats seem to be more supportive of anti-discrimination legislation than the Republicans.

418. Benjamin, A. E. and Philip R. Lee. "Public Policy, Federalism, and AIDS." <u>Death Studies</u>, v. 12, 1988, pp. 573-595.

AIDS presents a significant challenge to the American political system. The government response has been clouded by cutbacks in funding and uncertainty about the domain of issues surrounding AIDS. Stronger public leadership in the fight against AIDS is emerging.

419. Bethea, Dorine. "N.Y. Bills Touch AIDS/Uninsured." <u>National Underwriter (Life, Health, and Financial Services Edition)</u>, v. 92, August 22, 1988, pp. 4+.

The New York State Senate unanimously passed a bill that sets strict guidelines on the confidentiality of information related to patients with AIDS. However, doctors will be able to notify the sexual partners of an AIDS victim without the victim's consent.

420. Booth, William. "Congress Passes First AIDS Bill." <u>Science</u>, v. 242, October 21, 1988, p. 367.

In its first major response to the AIDS epidemic, Congress has passed a bill calling for AIDS education and prevention programs. The bill represents a compromise between liberal and conservative members and avoids the controversial subjects of AIDS testing and discrimination.

421. Colby, David C. and David G. Baker. "State Policy Responses to the AIDS Epidemic." <u>**Publius**</u>**, v. 18, Summer 1988, pp. 113-130.**

States have responded in a variety of ways to the AIDS epidemic. The degree and content of the legislation passed in each state is directly related to the incidence of the disease.

422. Colosi, Marco L. "AIDS: Human Rights Versus the Duty to Provide a Safe Workplace." <u>**Labor Law Journal**</u>**, v. 39, October 1988, pp. 677-687.**

Despite concerns about AIDS, the legal problems have yet to be resolved. The Centers for Disease Control has issued specific safety guidelines for employees in the health care occupations. Some of the legal implications of employees with AIDS in other industries are discussed.

423. Ehrlich, Elizabeth. "A Weapon That Could Backfire in the War on AIDS." <u>Business Week</u>, November 7, 1988, p. 92.

California voters will decide if people who are reasonably suspected of being infected by the AIDS virus should be required to be reported to public health officials. These persons would also be required to provide the state with a list of all of their sexual partners. This legislation would drive many infected persons underground, thus undermining the very reasons for its passage.

424. Eubanks, Paula. "States Have One Goal, Many Paths, to Fight AIDS." <u>Postgraduate Medicine</u>, v. 62, October 20, 1988, p. 68.

Each state has developed its own battle plan in the fight against AIDS. All states now require the reporting of AIDS cases, but they do not all require the reporting of the names of the patients. Legislators must be educated about AIDS so that they can pass meaningful AIDS legislation.

425. Field, Martha A. "Have Sex, Go to Jail." <u>Playboy</u>, v. 35, August 1988, pp. 34-35.

A man who is currently enlisted in military service has been charged with assault for having engaged in sex while knowingly infected by the AIDS virus. Some legislators are trying to make this and other actions of infected persons illegal.

426. Fumento, Michael J. "The Political Uses of an Epidemic." <u>New Republic</u>, v. 199, August 8, 1988, pp. 19-23.

Some conservatives are using AIDS to push for a new sexual morality. They would like to legislate against homosexuality and promiscuity. Most of this conservative agenda is based on a lack of knowledge about the disease.

427. Goerth, Charles R. "Restraining Order for Medical Insurance Urgent Attempt to Assist AIDS Victims." <u>Occupational Health and Safety</u>, v. 57, July 1988, p. 11.

The legal system has not handled enough AIDS cases to provide a clear ruling on AIDS discrimination cases. Many AIDS victims will die before their cases will be resolved. The case of an employer who dismissed an employee with AIDS is discussed.

428. Gregor, Anne. "Harsh Measures: The Dispute Over Tighter AIDS Regulations." <u>Maclean's</u>, v. 101, October 31, 1988, p. 55.

California voters will decide if the names of all persons with AIDS should be reported to state authorities. This proposition would also allow insurance companies to test applicants for antibodies to the AIDS virus. Critics argue that this legislation would violate the civil rights of AIDS victims and would be very costly to administer.

429. Haggerty, Alfred G. "AIDS Reporting Rejected By California Voters." <u>National Underwriter (Life, Health, and Financial Services Edition)</u>, v. 92, November 28, 1988, p. 19.

California voters soundly defeated a proposal to require the registration of persons reasonably believed to be infected by the AIDS virus. The initiative would also have required the reporting of all sexual partners of anyone testing positive for infection.

430. Holthaus, David. "Consent Advised Before AIDS Antibody Tests." <u>Hospitals</u>, v. 20, July 1988, pp. 40-42.

The testing of a hospital patient for AIDS without fist obtaining consent could be a liability time bomb for health care administrators. Patients who are tested without consent may later sue hospitals for negligence if this practice continues.

431. McFarren, Ann. "Help From the Top." <u>Christianity and Crisis</u>, v. 48, July 4, 1988, pp. 236-238.
     AIDS will be an important issue for the next president. The new administration must expand research programs and voluntary testing and counselling programs.

432. Mishkin, Douglas B. "Should Real Estate Professionals Disclose AIDS?" <u>Real Estate Today</u>, v. 21, November/December 1988, pp. 66-70.
     Although no medical evidence indicates that the AIDS virus can be transmitted through casual contact, real estate agents must decide if they should disclose whether any past residents of a house had AIDS. This information should not be disclosed. While the condition of the house is legally relevant to a sale, the condition of the owner is not.

433. "Out of Sight." <u>Economist</u>, v. 309, October 8, 1988, pp. 33-36.
     Neither presidential candidate has paid much attention to the issue of AIDS. Several political groups are trying a variety of tactics to make AIDS become a more visible part of the campaign.

434. Patner, Andrew. "AIDS Wasn't on the Agenda." <u>Progressive</u>, v. 52, October 1988, p. 12.
     Although over 39,000 people have died of AIDS, the Reagan administration has done very little to stop the spread of the disease. The Republican national convention approved a plank in its platform relating to AIDS, but it did not recommend increased funding or endorse the recommendations of the Presidential Commission on AIDS.

435. Pelosi, Nancy. "AIDS and Public Policy." <u>American Psychologist</u>, v. 43, November 1988, pp. 843-845.
     AIDS raises questions dealing with research priorities, prevention methods, and health care financing. The federal government must take the lead in the fight against the disease.

436. Rovner, Julie. "House Gears Up for Debate on AIDS Policy." <u>Congressional Quarterly Weekly Report</u>, v. 46, September 17, 1988, p. 2585.
     The House has set its ground rules for the first full debate on the topic of AIDS. This opens the door for the discussion and consideration of any AIDS-related legislation.

437. Rovner, Julie. "House Passes Bill Setting Federal AIDS Policy." <u>Congressional Quarterly Weekly Report</u>, v. 46, September 24, 1988, pp. 2652-2653.
     The House has passed the omnibus AIDS bill. Several amendments covering topics such as AIDS blood testing and the mandatory reporting of AIDS cases have been defeated. The Senate has already passed similar legislation and the bill will now go to a conference committee.

438. Rovner, Julie. "No Word From White House Yet on AIDS Bill." Congressional Quarterly Weekly Report, v. 46, October 22, 1988, pp. 3067-3071.
    The President has not yet signed the omnibus health bill on AIDS. Although the AIDS provisions have been carefully ironed out through compromises between conservative and liberal representatives, some of the non-AIDS portions of the bill may lead to its veto.

439. Rovner, Julie. "Omnibus Health Bill Cleared With Modified AIDS Provisions." Congressional Quarterly Weekly Report, v. 46, October 15, 1988, p. 2992.
    Congress has passed the first comprehensive health bill that discusses AIDS. However, planks dealing with confidentiality, testing, and discrimination had to be dropped in order to appease some conservative legislators.

440. Rovner, Julie. "Reagan Plan Dooms AIDS Anti-Bias Legislation." Congressional Quarterly Weekly Report, v. 46, August 6, 1988, p. 2189.
    The President's refusal to endorse legislation prohibiting discrimination against AIDS patients will probably kill all of the AIDS bills currently before Congress. Discrimination was one of the key points made by the Presidential Commission on AIDS, but it has been ignored by the President.

441. "Should HIV Carriers Have Secrets?" Time, v. 132, November 7, 1988, p. 36.
    California voters will decide whether persons testing positive for antibodies to the AIDS virus should be reported to the state. Under this legislation, anyone testing positive would also be required to provide a list of all of their sexual partners. Opponents see this proposal as discriminatory.

442. Street, John. "British Government Policy on AIDS: Learning Not to Die of Ignorance." Parliamentary Affairs, v. 41, October 1988, pp. 490-507.
    Presents the history of official government policy towards AIDS in Great Britain. The real substance of any AIDS policy is the amount of money it provides for research, treatment, education, and prevention. The government response in each of these areas is profiled.

443. United States. Congress. Senate. Committee on Government Affairs. Coordinating the Government's Response to AIDS: Health Care and Education. Washington, D.C.: Government Printing Office, 1988. 756p. Superintendent of Documents number Y4.G74/9:S.hrg.100-859.
    The full text of testimony examining the role of the federal government in stopping the spread of the AIDS virus. Government programs for health care and education are studied.

Discrimination Against AIDS Victims

444. Blendon, Robert J. and Karen Donelan. "Discrimination Against People With AIDS." <u>New England Journal of Medicine</u>, v. 319, October 13, 1988, pp. 1022-1026.

A survey was conducted to determine attitudes about AIDS and AIDS-related discrimination. Most agree that AIDS leads to discrimination, but they also believe that persons with AIDS should give up some of their civil rights. Public education alone will not stop discrimination. Additional legislation is needed.

445. Herek, Gregory M. and Eric K. Glunt. "An Epidemic of Stigma." <u>American Psychologist</u>, v. 43, November 1988, pp. 886-891.

The AIDS epidemic has generated a great deal of negative publicity about the groups of persons usually infected. This is the result of both identifying AIDS as a deadly and incurable disease and its association with socially stigmatized groups.

446. Poirier, Richard. "AIDS and Traditions of Homophobia." <u>Social Research</u>, v. 55, Autumn 1988, pp. 461-475.

Contemporary discourse on AIDS has increasingly become a moralistic condemnation of homosexuality. Such fears are not based on medical evidence, but on religious and social grounds. The AIDS epidemic is being used as a tool in the media war against homosexuality.

447. "Respect for AIDS Victims Rights, Wars Against Polio, Smoking Asked." <u>U.N. Chronicle</u>, v. 25, September 1988, pp. 66-67.

The United Nations has issued a call to all nations to avoid discrimination against AIDS victims. Governments should foster a spirit of understanding and compassion through information, education, and social support.

448. Rovner, Julie. "Justice Reverses AIDS Policy: Sen. Helms Delays Legislation." <u>Congressional Quarterly Weekly Report</u>, v. 46, October 8, 1988, p. 2810.

The Justice Department has reversed an earlier ruling that allowed discrimination against AIDS victims. The department now agrees that AIDS patients are protected under federal legislation designed to prevent discrimination against the handicapped. At the same time, conservative senators are attempting to block passage of additional AIDS legislation.

449. Sanders, Alain L. "Fighting AIDS Discrimination." <u>Time</u>, v. 132, September 5, 1988, p. 38.

A man who had been dropped from a Job Corps program because he tested positive for the AIDS virus has decided to file a lawsuit against the program. Many states have enacted legislation to prohibit such discrimination, but victims still have a long fight ahead.

AIDS and the Insurance Industry

450. "Actuaries Eye Up AIDS Victims." New Scientist, v. 119, July 14, 1988, p. 34.

The British insurance industry feels that all life insurance applicants should be tested for antibodies to the AIDS virus. The industry would like to include an automatic cancellation clause for anyone testing positive. It claims that this would save money for all policy holders.

451. "The AIDS Clause." Economist, v. 308, July 2, 1988, p. 14.

Insurance companies have long been trying to exclude coverage for persons infected by the AIDS virus. The flaws in the test methods make this process imprecise. Insurers should be allowed to use screening methods, but should be wary of test effectiveness.

452. "AIDS, Stress Claims Threaten Industry." National Underwriter (Property, Casualty, and Employee Benefits Edition), v. 92, September 12, 1988, pp. 52-53.

Insurance claims due to AIDS and stress may put a heavy financial burden on the insurance industry. By the year 2000, insurance companies are predicted to have paid out $50 billion for AIDS claims on life insurance policies that were already in effect before 1986.

453. Aldred, Carolyn. "AIDS Costs to Hit Various Nations Differently." Business Insurance, v. 22, September 26, 1988, p. 21.

AIDS will have different effects on insurance companies in different countries. AIDS claims will be much more easily absorbed into the mainstream insurance business in Europe than in either the United States or Great Britain.

454. Aldred, Carolyn. "AIDS Poses a Dilemma in the U.S." Business Insurance, v. 22, September 26, 1988, pp. 15-18.
State and federal laws are making it difficult for American insurance companies to reduce AIDS claims. Insurers cannot require applicants to be tested, cannot exclude coverage for AIDS and AIDS-related claims, and must pay for treatment with the drug zidovudine.

455. Aldred, Carolyn. "British Insurers Take Stand Against AIDS." Business Insurance, v. 22, September 26, 1988, pp. 14-15.

British insurers are taking all measures possible to protect themselves from AIDS claims. They are excluding coverage of AIDS, requiring AIDS blood tests, and increasing premiums for high-risk persons.

456. Arnold, Charles B., Stanley G. Karson, and Stephen D. Moskey. "International Conference Focuses on AIDS Woes." National Underwriter (Property, Casualty, and Employee Benefits Edition), v. 92, September 5, 1988, pp. 28-29. Also in National Underwriter (Life, Health, and Financial Services Edition), v. 92, September 5, 1988, pp. 14-15+.

   Three issues of interest to the insurance industry that were discussed at the Fourth International Conference on AIDS were the transmission and infectivity of the virus, behavior and risk education, and public policy. Many of these reports concentrated on the heterosexual spread of the virus.

457. Beal, Robert W. and Michael J. Cowell. "AIDS and Disability Insurance." Best's Review (Life/Health Insurance Edition), v. 89, October 1988, pp. 48-50+.

   In the next five years, 450,000 cases of AIDS have been projected. This could place a tremendous economic burden on the insurance industry. AIDS claims are more expensive than those for any other disease and could account for up to 25% of all expenses by the end of the century. The industry must be allowed to use screening in order to prevent economic disaster.

458. Bethea, Dorine. "U.K. Report Urges Exclusion Clause for HIV." National Underwriter (Life, Health, and Financial Services Edition), v. 92, September 26, 1988, pp. 6-7. Also in National Underwriter (Property, Casualty, and Employee Benefits Edition), v. 92, September 26, 1988, p. 113.

   A new report prepared by the British insurance industry recommends the use of exclusionary clauses for AIDS claims. The exclusionary clause on group policies would hold the employer responsible for AIDS claims rather than the insurer.

459. Connolly, Jim. "Dr. Defends AIDS Tests By Insurers." National Underwriter (Property, Casualty, and Employee Benefits Edition), v. 92, July 11, 1988, pp. 6+.

   A noted AIDS researcher believes that the insurance industry should be able to screen applicants to protect itself from AIDS claims. AIDS is an economic threat to the industry and testing provides a reasonable measure to prevent that threat.

460. "Counselling Caution." Economist, v. 308, August 6, 1988, pp. 47-48.

   Insurance companies have begun to classify everyone who has taken the AIDS test as a high risk, regardless of the outcome of that test. Others are requiring a negative test result before issuing a policy. Physicians feel that adequate counselling is not being given to persons who take the test for insurance purposes.

461. "Ethics and Transplants: Ethics and AIDS." <u>British Medical Journal</u>, v. 297, August 6, 1988, pp. 379-380.

The British Medical Association has protested the fact that insurance companies are testing applicants for AIDS infection. These objections are based on the fact that proper counselling is not provided with the tests.

462. Felter, Bethany. "Facing Up to the AIDS Threat." <u>**Best's Review (Life/Health Insurance Edition)**</u>**, v. 89, August 1988, pp. 142-144.**

AIDS has created a threatening mess for the insurance industry. Despite criticism, insurers do not feel that they have discriminated against anyone. In order to minimize costs, insurers should shift AIDS patients out of intensive care and into hospices or home care.

463. Grant, Daniel. "Health Insurance for Artists: The AIDS Stigma." <u>American Artist</u>, v. 52, July 1988, pp. 10+.

Insurance companies are classifying artists as a high risk group for AIDS. This concept is not stated explicitly, but it is obvious in their actions. The deaths of some prominent performing artists have created a negative stereotype of artists by insurers.

464. Haggerty, Alfred G. "Cal. Governor Expected to Sign AIDS Test Bill." <u>National Underwriter (Life, Health, and Financial Services Edition)</u>, v. 92, September 19, 1988, pp. 1+.

California has passed a bill allowing insurance companies to test applicants for infection by the AIDS virus. The insurance industry lobbied hard for the passage of this legislation.

465. Haggerty, Alfred G. "Expert Says: As Underwriting Goes, So Goes the Industry." <u>National Underwriter (Life, Health, and Financial Services Edition)</u>, v. 92, July 25, 1988, pp. 4+.

Bans on AIDS testing and the move towards unisex insurance may mean an end to the underwriting process. This could cause a fundamental change in the nature of the insurance industry.

466. Haggerty, Alfred G. "Life Executive Calls AIDS Threatening Mess." <u>National Underwriter (Life, Health, and Financial Services Edition)</u>, v. 92, July 25, 1988, pp. 4+.

AIDS is a dramatic economic problem for the insurance industry. Insurers must try to put caps on AIDS benefits and try to convince legislators that the disease will seriously hurt the industry.

467. "Health Insurers React to AIDS." <u>Accountancy</u>, v. 102, August 1988, p. 36.

Insurers offering permanent health insurance should consider excluding coverage of AIDS from their policies. A clause prohibiting payment for persons testing positive for the AIDS virus may protect companies from unusually high expenses.

468. Hiatt, Robert A. et al. <u>The Impact of AIDS on the Kaiser Permanente Medical Care Program (Northern Regional California)</u>. Washington, D.C.: Government Printing Office, July 1988. Office of Technology Assessment AIDS-Related Issues Series number 4. 45p. Superintendent of Documents number Y3.T22/2:Ac7/4.

From 1981 through June 1987, 940 members of one health insurance program were diagnosed as having AIDS. During this time, the rate of infection increased from 1.6 to 19.7 cases per 100,000 members. The median cost per case was estimated to be $29,929. The costs per case have been dropping over the last few years.

469. Huntley, Glenn. "Firm Suspends Policy Excluding AIDS Claims." <u>Business Insurance</u>, v. 22, August 15, 1988, pp. 2+.

One insurance company has dropped a policy that excluded coverage of AIDS, drug abuse, and other lifestyle-related claims. The company expected this policy to be controversial and eliminated it before any lawsuits were filed.

470. Ness, Immanuel. "AIDS Test Disclosure to MIB Rejected By NAIC Task Force." <u>National Underwriter (Life, Health, and Financial Services Edition)</u>, v. 92, December 19, 1988, pp. 1+.

A proposal to submit the results of all AIDS blood tests to a central database for use by the insurance industry has been rejected. The project was cancelled to protect the privacy of AIDS test results.

471. O'Hamilton, Joan and D. Castellon. "AIDS: Where Insurers Are Showing Little Mercy." <u>Business Week</u>, November 21, 1988, pp. 86-87.

Pressure from insurance companies to reduce AIDS claims is threatening small businesses. Some businesses change insurance companies every few years, leaving employees unprotected against any preexisting infections. Insurers are also dramatically raising rates for any companies who have employees with AIDS.

472. Taylor, Sebastian. "British Life Reinsurers Beef Up AIDS Reserves." <u>National Underwriter (Property, Casualty, and Employee Benefits Edition)</u>, v. 92, August 29, 1988, pp. 10-11. Also in <u>National Underwriter (Life, Health, and Financial Services Edition)</u>, v. 92, September 26, 1988, pp. 6-7+.

British reinsurers have been working to build up their financial reserves in order to protect themselves from AIDS claims. This reaction indicates either an alarmist response to AIDS in Britain or too lax a response in other nations.

473. "Truth in Insurance." _Fortune_, v. 118, September 26, 1988, p. 210.

The movement to ban insurance companies from testing applicants for infection by the AIDS virus is losing its steam. Three states and the District of Columbia have passed such legislation, but in all four cases the legislation is being challenged by the insurance industry.

474. United States. Office of Technology Assessment. _Medical Testing and Health Insurance_. Washington, D.C.: Government Printing Office, 1988. 35p. Superintendent of Documents number Y3.T22/2:2M46/11/sum.

The concept of underwriting is commonly used to determine the insurability of individual applicants who have preexisting conditions that indicate a higher risk of disease. Insurance companies would like to use the AIDS blood test to screen for persons infected by the AIDS virus. The exclusion of AIDS patients from private insurance policies could put a greater burden on government health care programs.

The Costs of the AIDS Epidemic

475. Andrews, Roxanne M., Margaret A. Keyes, and Penelope L. Pine. "Acquired Immunodeficiency Syndrome in California's Medicaid Program, 1981-1984." <u>Health Care Financing Review</u>, v. 10, Fall 1988, pp. 95-103.

The cost of AIDS to the California Medicaid program was calculated. Expenditures increased during the first two years of the study, but decreased during the third. This decrease was due to a change in hospital reimbursement methods and not to a decline in the number of hospital stays.

476. Benjamin, A. E. "Long-Term Care and AIDS: Perspective From Experience With the Elderly." <u>Milbank Quarterly</u>, v. 66, 1988, pp. 415-443.

Cost containment measures for AIDS have concentrated on minimizing hospital care. Experiences with the elderly indicate that this procedure produces a greater impact on all services while not really reducing costs. Medical care should play a central role in the management of AIDS.

477. Black, G. J., Jr. "AIDS Care: Ingredient for Financial Disaster or Decision?" <u>Healthcare Financial Management</u>, v. 42, November 1988, p. 10.

AIDS is placing a great deal of pressure on the already overburdened health care financing industry. AIDS costs may reach $8.5 billion by 1991. Hospitals must work to reduce the costs of AIDS cases while still protecting both patients and employees.

478. Cella, Margot and D. Earl Brown, Jr. "AIDS Treatment a Financial Burden for Hospitals, Other Providers." <u>Healthcare Financial Management</u>, v. 42, November 1988, pp. 52-58.

The cost of AIDS averages $35,461 per case for adults and $53,574 per case for children. Most of these expenses are covered by health insurance, but expenditures for medicaid programs for AIDS patients reached $400 million in 1987. These costs will only increase as the number of cases increases.

479. Ford, Peter and David Robertson. "AIDS and the Small City: The Cost at Kingston General Hospital." <u>Canadian Medical Association Journal</u>, v. 139, September 15, 1988, pp. 557-562.

AIDS is becoming a serious issue for physicians and hospitals in small cities. The cost of AIDS to a hospital in such a city is estimated to be $700,000. AIDS also requires a larger investment of labor than most other diseases.

480. Gomez, Michael. "Managing Healthcare Costs: The Dilemma of AIDS." Compensation and Benefits Review, v. 20, September/October 1988, pp. 23-31.
     The costs of AIDS care can be reduced through individual case management. Before this occurs, employers, insurers, and the public need to learn how to deal with the disease rationally.

481. Haggerty, Alfred G. "Calif. Health Plan Projects $88M AIDS Price Tag." National Underwriter (Life, Health, and Financial Services Edition), v. 92, August 22, 1988, pp. 11+.
     One California insurer expects to pay out $87.7 million for AIDS claims by 1990. A total of 940 members of the program have already been diagnosed with AIDS. The average lifetime cost of the disease has been estimated at $35,054.

482. Hegarty, James D. et al. "The Medical Care Costs of Human Immunodeficiency Virus-Infected Children in Harlem." JAMA: Journal of the American Medical Association, v. 260, October 7, 1988, pp. 1901-1905.
     The medical care costs of 37 children at a New York hospital were calculated. The average lifetime cost was determined to be $90,347 per child. Costs were highest for those children suffering from opportunistic infections and lowest for "boarder babies" who had no home to which they could be returned.

483. Hellinger, Fred J. "National Forecasts of the Medical Care Costs of AIDS: 1988-1992." Inquiry, v. 25, Winter 1988, pp. 469-484.
     Using a statistical model, forecasts are made on the costs of individual AIDS cases over the next four years. The number of cases is expected to be higher than originally predicted, but the cost of a single case should be lower. The lifetime cost of treating all AIDS victims could reach $6 billion by 1992.

484. "Individual AIDS Care Costs Decreasing Over Time, Study Shows." American Pharmacy, v. 28, December 1988, p. 17.
     The cost of treating AIDS patients is less than previously estimated. A new study showed an average lifetime hospital cost for AIDS of $27,264. This is significantly lower than the $42,000 to $147,000 range reported earlier.

485. Lafferty, William E. et al. "Hospital Charges for People With AIDS in Washington State: Utilization of a Statewide Hospital Discharge Data Base." American Journal of Public Health, v. 78, August 1988, pp. 949-952.
     In Washington, the mean charge for hospitalization of AIDS patients was $9,166 and the mean length of stay was 13.3 days. AIDS hospitalizations are substantially more expensive than those for other diseases.

486. Robinson, Michele L. and Alden T. Solovy. "Kaiser Emphasizes Outpatient Care for AIDS." Hospitals, v. 62, August 20, 1988, p. 42.

By moving AIDS patients to outpatient care, one hospital has reduced its cost per patient by over one-third. This was made possible by using the existing social services within the community to provide much of the care.

487. Seage, George R., III, et al. "Medical Costs of Ambulatory Patients with the AIDS-Related Complex (ARC) and/or Generalized Lymphadenopathy Syndrome (GLS) Related to HIV Infection, 1984-95." American Journal of Public Health, v. 78, August 1988, pp. 969-970.

A cost of illness study was conducted on 28 patients with the AIDS-related complex or generalized lymphadenopathy syndrome. The average cost was $489 per patient per year. None of the patients in the study required hospitalization or treatment with zidovudine.

488. United States. Congress. Senate. Committee on Finance. Subcommittee on Social Security and Family Policy. Social Security Benefits for AIDS Victims. Washington, D.C.: Government Printing Office, 1988. 119p. Superintendent of Documents number Y4.F49:S.hrg.100-645.

The complete text of a Senate hearing on social security benefits for AIDS patients. The availability of benefits, the impact of AIDS on the social security system, and the special needs of children with AIDS are all discussed.

489. West, Peter A. "The Cost of AIDS: Discussion Paper." Journal of the Royal Society of Medicine, v. 81, September 1988, pp. 540-541.

AIDS has caused high costs in both human suffering and economics. If 5,000 cases per year are reported in Britain, the total cost will be 135 million pounds. Such cost estimates are not worth making because they are highly uncertain, they include very high drug costs, they do not take into account the services provided, and they draw an unwanted scrutiny to the fight against the disease.

Funding for AIDS Research

490. Booth, William. "No Longer Ignored." <u>Science</u>, v. 242, November 11, 1988, pp. 858-859.

After being underfunded for several years, AIDS programs are now reaching the same funding levels as those for cancer and heart disease. AIDS funding is becoming the major source of income for some agencies and AIDS funding is beginning to support research in other areas.

491. Eubanks, Paula. "Hospitals Seek Philanthropists to Fight AIDS." <u>Hospitals</u>, v. 62, December 5, 1988, p. 24.

Many private foundations are donating more money for AIDS research and treatment than they have in the past, but they cannot meet all of the current demands. Some foundations are also now directly funding grass-roots AIDS organizations.

492. "Spend More on AIDS Research, Ottawa Advised." <u>Canadian Medical Association Journal</u>, v. 139, December 15, 1988, p. 1181.

The Canadian government intends to spend $129 million on AIDS over the next five years, but none of this funding will be targeted for basic research. Some researchers feel that this figure is inadequate.

493. Sun, Marjorie. "NIH Budget Boost Mostly for AIDS." <u>Science</u>, v. 241, September 16, 1988, p. 1427.

The budget for the National Institutes of Health will increase 7% in 1989 to over $7.1 billion. Most of this increase will be used to fund AIDS research.

494. United States. Congress. House. <u>AIDS Research Act of 1988</u>. Washington, D.C.: Government Printing Office, 1988. 38p. Superintendent of Documents number Y1.1/8:100-815.

A report supporting the passage of the AIDS Research Act of 1988. This act proposes the allocation of additional funding and personnel to be used in the fight against the disease.

AIDS and the Media

495. **Colen, B. D.** **"Paying the Price of AIDS."** <u>Health</u>, v. 20, October 1988, pp. 32+.

Media coverage of AIDS has declined as writers have become tired of the disease. The majority of readers have also become disinterested because AIDS is a disease primarily infecting other groups of people. However, everyone will soon carry the economic burden of the disease.

496. Coles, Peter. "Five Years of French AIDS Coverage." <u>Nature</u>, v. 336, November 3, 1988, p. 8.

Media coverage of the AIDS epidemic has revolutionized the image of the scientist for the general public. However, the media is beginning to lose interest in AIDS. Only a significant breakthrough will bring AIDS back into the forefront of media coverage.

497. Connor, Steve. "U.S. Seeks to Suppress Publication in Europe of AIDS Book." <u>New Scientist</u>, v. 120, December 17, 1988, pp. 8-9.

The United States government is attempting to stop the publication of a new book on the discovery of the AIDS virus. The government claims that the book is full of scientific errors and false statements. This action is being taken as a form of censorship by European publishers.

498. "Does Safe Sex Sell?" <u>Glamour</u>, v. 86, July 1988, p. 156.

Although safe sex has been a topic of discussion on television, it is not a standard practice of characters in films. Directors have not changed the sexual behaviors of their characters because they do not believe that audiences want to see films about AIDS.

499. Grube, Anette and Karin Boehme-Duerr. "AIDS in International News Magazines." <u>Journalism Quarterly</u>, v. 65, Fall 1988, pp. 686-689.

The coverage of AIDS was studied in five international news magazines. No direct relationship was found between the number of AIDS cases within a country and the coverage of the disease by that nation's media.

500. Kemp, Jim. "Normalizing an Epidemic." <u>Christianity and Crisis</u>, v. 48, July 4, 1988, pp. 227-229.

The media has concentrated on AIDS as the gay plague and has blamed the victims for their own illness. Even programs that warn that everyone is at risk for AIDS carry a subtle blame of the high risk groups. The vocabulary used to describe AIDS must be changed in order to avoid a confrontational attitude.

501. Laermer, Richard. "High School Journalists Help Battle AIDS." <u>Editor and Publisher</u>, v. 121, August 20, 1988, p. 18.

The Red Cross has held a conference on AIDS for high school journalists. The purpose of this conference was to get high school students interested in educating their peers about the disease.

502. "Media Are Losing Interest in AIDS." <u>Editor and Publisher</u>, v. 121, November 5, 1988, p. 18.

After running many human interest stories about AIDS, the media seem to be losing interest in the disease. The next big push for media interest will occur when a cure is discovered.

503. Meyers, Janet. "Dilemma Over Paid AIDS Ads." <u>Advertising Age</u>, v. 59, October 31, 1988, p. 41.

Congress has authorized $45 million for a national AIDS advertising campaign. Some officials fear that the use of paid advertising will cause some stations to drop the free public service announcements about AIDS that are currently being used.

504. Murphy, Mary. "The AIDS Scare: What It's Done to Hollywood and the TV You See." <u>TV Guide</u>, v. 36, October 22, 1988, pp. 4-9.

Although outwardly Hollywood has led the fight against AIDS, the attitude inside the film industry has become very restrictive. Men are no longer free to admit their homosexuality for fear of losing their jobs due to a fear of AIDS.

The Presidential Commission on AIDS

505. "AIDS Commission Issues Report: Gets Lukewarm Response."
<u>American Pharmacy</u>, v. 28, November 1988, pp. 19-21.
    The Presidential Commission on AIDS has issued its final
report, which includes nearly 600 recommendations for action.
Many of these recommendations are highlighted.

506. "AIDS: Taking Action." <u>National Review</u>, v. 40, July 8,
1988, pp. 17-18.
    None of the proposals made by the Presidential Commission
on AIDS takes us any closer to finding a cure for the disease.
The recommendations try to provide a humanitarian environment
for dealing with AIDS, but they only limit the rights of
employers and individuals.

507. "A Blueprint for Change: What's Ahead for Nursing in the
Age of AIDS?" <u>Nursing 88</u>, v. 18, August 1988, pp. 28-29.
    The proposals made by the President's Commission on AIDS
could have wide-ranging effects on the nursing and health care
professions. Several of the commission's recommendations are
highlighted.

508. Booth, William. "AIDS Report Draws Tepid Response."
<u>Science</u>, v. 241, August 12, 1988, p. 778.
    President Reagan has called for two studies in response
to the final report of the Presidential Commission on AIDS.
Critics feel that he should have reacted more strongly to the
recommendations of the commission.

509. Ezzell, Carol. "Compromise Report Issued By White House
AIDS Commission." <u>Nature</u>, v. 334, July 7, 1988, p. 7.
    The final report of the Presidential Commission on AIDS
has been released. It does not appear that the White House
will move quickly in responding to the recommendations made
by this report.

510. Kerr, Diane L. "Presidential Commission Report on the
HIV Epidemic." <u>Journal of School Health</u>, v. 58, September
1988, p. 306.
    The final report of the Presidential Commission on AIDS
calls for school-based AIDS education programs. In the short
term, schools should integrate appropriate information on AIDS
into the curriculum. In the long term, schools should develop
comprehensive school health programs.

**511. Marwick, Charles. "Follow-Up Report on AIDS Commission
Recommendations Goes to President Soon." <u>JAMA: Journal of the
American Medical Association</u>, v. 260, September 9, 1988, pp.
1340-1345.**
    A ten point action plan has been developed by the White
House in response to the Presidential Commission on AIDS, but
it has come under fire as too weak by some groups. The most
disappointing aspect of this plan is the lack of support for
antidiscrimination and confidentiality measures.

512. Marwick, Charles. "White House Aide Studying AIDS Commission Recommendations: Reports to President Soon." JAMA: Journal of the American Medical Association, v. 260, August 5, 1988, p. 602.

The President has directed the White House's special assistant for drug policy to review the recommendations made by the Presidential Commission on AIDS. The proposals that have created some controversy are those that deal with the confidentiality of test results and those that attempt to reduce the bureaucracy of the National Institutes of Health.

513. **Marwick, Charles and Phil Gunby. "AIDS Recommendations Leave Federal Officials to Ponder: Where Do We Go From Here?" JAMA: Journal of the American Medical Association, v. 260, July 1, 1988, pp. 16-17.**

The final report of the Presidential Commission on AIDS calls for a major restructuring of the health care system. The 580 recommendations made by the report cover a wide range of issues, including drug abuse, patient care, and AIDS treatments. The report also calls for new legislation to protect confidentiality and to prevent discrimination.

514. "More Missed Chances." Nature, v. 334, August 11, 1988, p. 457.

President Reagan has failed to implement the recommendations of his own commission on AIDS. He did not want to endorse the antidiscrimination concerns of the report. The next President will have to act quickly to avoid an even greater epidemic.

515. "Report of the Presidential Commission on the Human Immunodeficiency Virus Epidemic." Journal of School Health, v. 58, October 1988, pp. 327-329.

A summary of the recommendations made by the Presidential Commission on AIDS. School-based education programs will be critical in stopping the spread of the disease.

516. Watkins, James D. "Responding to the HIV Epidemic." American Psychologist, v. 43, November 1988, pp. 849-851.

The Presidential Commission on AIDS has issued a report containing hundreds of recommendations for stopping the spread of the AIDS virus. More funding for AIDS is needed and an increased emphasis should be placed on behavioral research.

The People of the AIDS Epidemic

517. Armstrong, Sallie. "When AIDS Strikes Close to Home." Parents' Magazine, v. 63, September 1988, pp. 85-88.

The story of how one family reacted to a neighbor's death from AIDS. Initial fear and rejection of the victim's family were replaced by understanding after attending an AIDS education seminar.

518. Bass, Thomas. "Luc Montagnier." Omni, v. 11, December 1988, pp. 102-104+.

An interview with Dr. Luc Montagnier, the first researcher to isolate the AIDS virus.

519. Berrigan, Daniel. "Luke's Passage: In the Evening We Will Be Judged By Love." U.S. Catholic, v. 53, November 1988, pp. 30-36.

The story of a priest who ministered to a patient with AIDS. The priest learned that even those who are down and out can still be happy if they are filled with love.

520. Brodsley, Laurel. "A Freshman English Class Talks About Sex, Risk Taking, and AIDS." Journal of Sex Research, v. 25, August 1988, pp. 433-436.

A group of college students discuss their feelings about AIDS. Most do not want to engage in safe sex and feel that AIDS will not affect them.

521. Conniff, Richard. "Families That Open Their Homes to the Sick." Time, v. 132, December 5, 1988, pp. 12-14.

Several foster families that take in children with AIDS are profiled. Foster parents of children with AIDS run the extra risk of loving children who will either be taken away from them or die.

522. DeWolfe, Mark M. "Love and Let Love." Christianity and Crisis, v. 48, July 4, 1988, pp. 221-223.

A Unitarian minister recounts his ordeal with AIDS. He had to re-learn how to interact with his congregation after he learned that he had the disease.

523. Edwards, Owen. "Mortal Vision." American Photographer, v. 21, December 1988, pp. 18-20.

A photographer has opened an exhibition of photographs of AIDS victims. These photographs can teach viewers more about the suffering caused by the disease than many of the existing AIDS education programs.

524. Elliott, Deni. "Identifying AIDS Victims." WJR: Washington Journalism Review, v. 10, October 1988, pp. 26-29.

The story of a pediatrician who had tested positive for AIDS. Once this fact became known through a local court case, the media picked up the story and he lost most of his patients to fears about the disease.

525. "Farewell Gift." Life, v. 11, November 1988, p. 52.
     An AIDS patient who worked on pipe organs was looking for
a job to boost his morale. A church in San Francisco gave him
the opportunity to restore its old pipe organ. This organ
will remain as his legacy long after his death.

526. "Fauci, Anthony Stephen." Current Biography Yearbook,
v. 49, 1988, pp. 153-156.
     A biography of the director of AIDS research at the
National Institutes of Health.

527. Fredericks, Ann. "The Baby Nobody Wanted." Ladies Home
Journal, v. 105, September 1988, pp. 22-24.
     The story of a foster family who took in an infant with
AIDS. Although extra precautions are required, caring for a
child with AIDS is a joy.

528. Fuchs, Elinor. "The AIDS Quilt." Nation, v. 247,
October 31, 1988, pp. 408-409.
     The AIDS Quilt Project was conducted as a memorial to
those who have died of the disease. Each of the over 8,000
panels was made out of love for an individual. The quilt is
a symbol of the struggle to fight the disease.

529. Goldstein, William. "Paul Monette Reflects on AIDS and
His Own Borrowed Time." Publishers Weekly, v. 234, December
2, 1988, pp. 19-20.
     A new book portrays the death of the author's lover from
AIDS. The book attempts to provide a personal account of both
the suffering and the love involved in the relationship.

530. Grady, Denise. "AIDS Survivors." American Health, v.
7, September 1988, pp. 78-85.
     A few AIDS victims live with the disease for a much
longer period of time than average. It is possible that AIDS
may not be 100% fatal. Studies of these long-term survivors
may yield clues that can be used in fighting the disease.

531. "HHS Honors RNs As Unsung Heroes in AIDS Fight."
American Journal of Nursing, v. 88, October 1988, pp. 1422+.
     Working with AIDS patients is heart-warming and reminds
nurses why they entered into the profession. Several nurses
have been rewarded for their outstanding care of AIDS
patients.

532. Jackson, Michael S. and Gail Hovey. "Fighting AIDS on
the Streets." Christianity and Crisis, v. 48, July 4, 1988,
pp. 238-240.
     An interview with the head of an AIDS prevention
organization. This group works to stop the spread of AIDS
among drug users.

533. Johnson, Bonnie. "California's Starcross Community Helps the Littlest Victims of AIDS Savor Life in the Shadow of Death." People, v. 30, December 12, 1988, pp. 152-156.

A Catholic order in California has established a home that cares for children with AIDS. The local community was fearful of the program at first, but has since learned that there is no danger of transmission of the virus.

534. Lewis, Angie. "Development of AIDS Awareness: A Personal History." Death Studies, v. 12, 1988, pp. 371-379.

A nurse who worked closely with AIDS patients learned new truths about herself, her colleagues, and her community. Some of the personal challenges that AIDS presents to nurses are discussed.

535. Mandell, Harvey N. "AIDS: A Patient's View." Postgraduate Medicine, v. 84, September 1, 1988, pp. 36-38.

Much research has been done about the medical and scientific aspects of AIDS. However, there are very few reports from patients on what it is like to have the disease. An AIDS patient is interviewed about his personal reactions to the disease.

536. Masson, Veneta. "Facing AIDS." Nursing Outlook, v. 36, September/October 1988, p. 225.

The story of how AIDS has affected an inner-city neighborhood. Nurses working in such areas need to offer hope to their patients because they will not find it anywhere else.

537. "Montagnier, Luc." Current Biography Yearbook, v. 49, 1988, pp. 402-405.

A biography of the French scientist who was the first to isolate the AIDS virus.

538. Newman, Frank. "Aids, Youth, and the University." Change, v. 20, September/October 1988, pp. 39-44.

An interview with the chair of the Presidential Commission on AIDS. Education is our primary weapon for controlling the spread of the disease.

539. Novicki, Margaret A. "Dr. Mathilde Krim: Waging War Against AIDS." Africa Report, v. 33, November/December 1988, pp. 23-25.

An interview with Dr. Mathilde Krim, one of the world's most prominent AIDS researchers. The heterosexual nature of AIDS in Africa, the origins of the virus, and the economic impact of AIDS are all discussed.

540. Oyler, Chris. "Go Toward the Light." Reader's Digest, v. 133, November 1988, pp. 207-260.

The story of a couple who had a child who died of AIDS. The child was a hemophiliac who contracted the disease through blood transfusions.

541. "Playboy Interview: Harvey Fierstein." Playboy, v. 35, August 1988, pp. 43-53.
     AIDS has changed the lifestyle of homosexuals in the United States. A leader in the homosexual community discusses life under the threat of AIDS.

542. Rosellini, Lynn. "The Metamorphosis of the AIDS Admiral." U.S. News and World Report, v. 105, July 4, 1988, p. 30.
     A profile of James D. Watkins, the chair of the Presidential Commission on AIDS. While starting out as a hard line conservative, his experience with the commission quickly turned him into an advocate for persons with the disease.

543. "Salute to Courage." Saturday Evening Post, v. 260, September 1988, pp. 12+.
     Dr. Edgar G. Engleman was the first person to screen donated blood for contamination by the AIDS virus. This procedure has since become standard practice and has prevented the further spread of AIDS through the blood supply.

544. SerVaas, Cory. "AIDS Patient Warns Others." Saturday Evening Post, v. 260, July/August 1988, pp. 98-100.
     The story of an elderly woman who contracted AIDS from her husband, who had become infected through a blood transfusion. She recommends that people store their own blood for later use to prevent infection.

545. Shapiro, Harriet. "Facing Down Her Fears About AIDS Was a Risk-Filled Act for Novelist Alice Hoffman." People, v. 30, September 12, 1988, pp. 101-103.
     A new novel tells the story of a family that must confront a child who contracted AIDS through a blood transfusion. The author often wonders how she would react to AIDS in her own family.

546. "Soldier in the War Against AIDS." Black Enterprise, v. 19, October 1988, p. 62.
     A profile of Dr. Helane D. Gayle, an epidemiologist who is working to help stop the spread of AIDS. Hard work will be required, but there is hope for an end to the disease.

547. Springs, John B., III. "AIDS: Yes or No?" Essence, v. 19, November 1988, p. 8.
     The story of a prison inmate who asked to be tested for infection by the AIDS virus. The reaction of the prison system was one of fear and rejection until the negative test results were received.

548. Trent, Bill. "A Place for Living, a Place for Dying."
<u>Canadian Medical Association Journal</u>, v. 139, November 1,
1988, pp. 889-893.
     A shelter for AIDS patients is profiled. All of the
residents know that they are going to die from the disease,
but they come to this hospice for a sense of community during
their last days.

549. Verber, I. "It Is Not One of Them, It Is One of All of
Us." <u>British Medical Journal</u>, v. 297, July 9, 1988, p. 149.
     The story of one man's ordeal with a friend who had AIDS.
It is only when the disease strikes close to home that one
realizes the enormity of the AIDS problem.

550. Woody, John. "My Brother Was a Person. He Also Had
AIDS." <u>RN</u>, v. 51, December 1988, p. 102.
     A nurse whose brother died of AIDS has come to view the
disease differently because of this personal experience.
Watching a person suffer can help remove the labels of guilt
often associated with AIDS.

The Worldwide AIDS Epidemic

551. "AIDS Update." <u>British Medical Journal</u>, v. 297, October 22, 1988, p. 1003.

As of September 1988, 1,794 cases of AIDS have been reported in Great Britain and 965 of those victims have died. The distribution of these cases among the various risk groups is presented.

552. Armstrong, Sue. "Fear and Ignorance in the Arab World." <u>New Scientist</u>, v. 119, September 1, 1988, p. 37.

In Arab societies, AIDS is seen as punishment from God for immoral acts. AIDS education is much more difficult to carry out in this environment of ignorance and denial.

553. Barry, Michele. "Ethical Considerations of Human Investigation in Developing Countries." <u>New England Journal of Medicine</u>, v. 319, October 20, 1988, pp. 1083-1086.

Considerations must be made of the ethical and cultural factors involved in studying large populations of AIDS victims in Third World nations. Participation in studies must be voluntary, no harm must be done to the subjects, the benefits and burdens of research must be distributed fairly, and the research must be carefully reviewed by outside governing bodies.

554. Bazell, Robert. "A Third-World Scourge." <u>Discover</u>, v. 9, September 1988, pp. 16-18.

Although AIDS may be restricted to high risk groups in the United States, it is realizing epidemic proportions among Third World nations. In some countries, such as Haiti, cultural traditions tend to encourage the spread of the disease. Some parts of Africa have literally been decimated by the disease.

555. Bonneux, Luc et al. "Risk Factors for Infection with Human Immunodeficiency Virus Among European Expatriates in Africa." <u>British Medical Journal</u>, v. 297, September 3, 1988, pp. 581-584.

The pattern of AIDS infection in Belgium suggests that Europeans initially acquired the virus in Africa. Approximately 1% of the Europeans living in Africa tested positive for the virus. Infected men outnumbered women three to one, but the subjects were not drug users or homosexuals. Sexual contact with local women or prostitutes and injections by unqualified medical staff were the highest risk factors for infection.

556. Chikwem, John O. et al. "Impact of Health Education on Prostitutes' Awareness and Attitudes to Acquired Immune Deficiency Syndrome (AIDS)." Public Health, v. 102, September 1988, pp. 439-445.

A survey was conducted to determine AIDS awareness among African prostitutes. Most prostitutes seem to be receptive to AIDS education programs. They also advocate restrictions on persons who are infected by the AIDS virus.

557. Christakis, Nicholas A. "The Ethical Design of an AIDS Vaccine Trial in Africa." Hastings Center Report, v. 18, June/July 1988, pp. 31-37.

Vaccine trials should take into account the ethical and social values of the nation in which the trials occur. The concept of informed consent must be adapted to fit African society. The risks and benefits of medical developments must also be viewed differently in nations with limited resources.

558. Clifford, M. "Letter From Seoul." Far Eastern Economic Review, v. 142, October 27, 1988, p. 110.

South Koreans view AIDS as a scourge brought to their country by foreigners. Some are using AIDS as a reason to require the expulsion of American military personnel.

559. Coles, Peter. "Concern Mounting Over French Government Action on AIDS." Nature, v. 335, September 22, 1988, p. 290.

Public concern is mounting over the French government's response to AIDS. Three distinguished doctors have called for additional testing to determine the extent of the epidemic.

560. Coles, Peter. "Coordination Is the Key for New AIDS Research Programme." Nature, v. 336, December 8, 1988, p. 508.

The French AIDS program is going to emphasize coordinated research and international cooperation. The budget for basic research has been doubled and three million francs have been allocated for studies on the sociology of the disease.

561. Coles, Peter. "French Government Recognizes Need for AIDS Health Campaign." Nature, v. 335, September 1, 1988, p. 2.

France has the highest per capita incidence of AIDS outside of the United States. An AIDS education campaign is needed and a special effort must be made to inform drug users about the risks of infection.

562. Coles, Peter. "Long-Awaited French Anti-AIDS Campaign Is Launched." Nature, v. 336, November 10, 1988, p. 98.

The French government is increasing its efforts against AIDS. The budget for AIDS research grants has been tripled and the budget for AIDS education has been increased by a factor of four.

563. Coles, Peter. "Proposed AIDS Screening Causes Political Turmoil in France." Nature, v. 334, August 11, 1988, p. 461.
A plan for widespread screening of pregnant women for infection by the AIDS virus has led to the resignation of a French health official. This reinforces the fact that AIDS is a political as well as a medical problem.

564. Connor, Steve and Sharon Kingman. "AIDS Cases Set to Grow Fifteenfold." New Scientist, v. 120, December 3, 1988, pp. 23-24.
Projections indicate that the number of AIDS cases in Britain will increase by a factor of fifteen over the next four years. The number of heterosexually transmitted cases remains unclear because sexual behaviors of heterosexuals have yet to change due to AIDS.

565. Dickman, Steven. "Bavarian AIDS Ruling Will Go to Appeal." Nature, v. 334, July 14, 1988, p. 94.
It may be difficult to prosecute persons who knowingly transmit the AIDS virus in Bavaria. Prosecution can only take place when the recipient actually develops AIDS, which can be many years after the act of transmission of the virus.

566. Dickson, David. "France Boosts AIDS Funds." Science, v. 242, November 11, 1988, p. 862.
The French government has finally increased its support for AIDS research. Funding levels in France will now be equivalent to those of Great Britain and West Germany.

567. Dickson, David. "France Failing to Build on Early AIDS Research?" Science, v. 242, October 28, 1988, pp. 509-510.
Although France was the first nation in which the AIDS virus was isolated, it does not have a long-term AIDS policy. Critics feel that AIDS research in France has already fallen behind that of other nations.

568. Dorozyneski, Alexander. "French AIDS Register." British Medical Journal, v. 297, October 22, 1988, pp. 1003-1004.
French health officials are planning to establish a national register of persons who have been infected by the AIDS virus. A computer code will protect the anonymity of persons listed in this database.

569. Ezzell, Carol. "Still No Government Reply to Canada's AIDS Report." Nature, v. 335, September 1, 1988, p. 2.
The Canadian government has yet to respond to a report on the incidence of AIDS, despite the fact that Canada has one of the highest levels of infection in the world. The government is allocating $52 million for AIDS education and is making this one of its top priorities.

570. Gallup, George, Jr. and Alec M. Gallup. "AIDS: 35-Nation Survey." Gallup Report, no. 273, June 1988, pp. 2-73.
     The results of an international poll on AIDS awareness. Although the knowledge level about the disease is high, not enough people are changing their behaviors to avoid the transmission of the virus.

571. "A Global Response to AIDS." Africa Report, v. 33, November/December 1988, pp. 13-16.
     AIDS has hit sub-Saharan Africa especially hard and is most severe in central and eastern Africa. The vast majority of African cases involve heterosexual transmission of the virus. The World Health Organization is working to stop the spread of the disease worldwide.

572. Goldsmith, Marsha F. "Africa Says It's Not Too Late As Fight Against AIDS Intensifies." JAMA: Journal of the American Medical Association, v. 260, September 2, 1988, pp. 1193-1198.
     After nearly a decade of denial, African nations are now beginning to react to the crisis of AIDS. One of the most pressing needs in Africa is the establishment of a safe blood supply. Efforts are also under way to increase condom usage, especially with prostitutes.

573. Gunson, H. H. and V. I. Rawlinson. "AIDS Update." British Medical Journal, v. 297, July 23, 1988, p. 244.
     As of June 1988, 1,598 cases of AIDS had been reported in Great Britain and 897 of these victims have died. Only 92 of nearly six million blood donors have tested positive for AIDS infection.

574. Hilts, Philip J. "Dispelling Myths About AIDS in Africa." Africa Report, v. 33, November/December 1988, pp. 26-31.
     AIDS is a substantial problem for only a few of the 53 African nations. The disease is clustered in urban areas and along highways, but most rural areas remain unaffected. Health officials are also angered that some scientists claim that AIDS originated in Africa.

575. Katzin, Louise. "AIDS Cases Worldwide." American Journal of Nursing, v. 88, September 1988, p. 1172.
     As of July 1988, over 100,000 cases of AIDS have been reported worldwide. Three-fourths of all cases are found in the Americas, 12% in Africa, 13% in Europe, and less than 1% in the rest of the world.

576. Kingman, Sharon. "Genital Ulcers Promote Spread in Africa." New Scientist, v. 119, September 22, 1988, pp. 28-29.
     African men who had genital ulcers were much more likely to become infected with the AIDS virus than men in other categories. Genital ulcers could be an important cofactor in the spread of the virus in Africa.

577. Kingman, Sharon. "Ten Times More AIDS Cases in Africa." New Scientist, v. 119, September 22, 1988, p. 20.

The World Health Organization suspects that the actual number of cases of AIDS in Africa is ten times the number that have been reported. Zaire has reported no new cases since the 335 reported as of June 1987, yet a computer model projects that the nation probably has had at least 50,000 new cases. More accurate data are needed about the spread of AIDS in Africa.

578. Losos, Joseph et al. "Acquired Immune Deficiency Syndrome in Canada: The First Five Years of Surveillance." Canadian Medical Association Journal, v. 139, September 1, 1988, pp. 383-388.

Over 1,100 cases of AIDS have been reported in Canada since 1982. Over 82% of these cases were among homosexual or bisexual men. Geographically, British Columbia, Quebec, and Ontario represent almost 90% of all Canadian cases.

579. Mann, Jonathan M. "AIDS: A Global Strategy for a Global Challenge." Impact of Science on Society, no. 150, 1988, pp. 159-167.

AIDS is becoming one of the greatest medical challenges of our century. The virus has been found in nearly every nation and it is causing social and political concerns as well as becoming a significant medical problem. Only an international program to fight this disease will stop its further spread.

580. Mann, Jonathan M. and James Chin. "AIDS: A Global Perspective." New England Journal of Medicine, v. 319, August 4, 1988, pp. 302-303.

As of July 1, 1988, over 100,000 cases of AIDS have been reported to the World Health Organization. Transmission of the virus occurs through blood, sex, and pregnancy. Three distinct patterns of infection have been determined, each of which occurs in a different geographic area. A worldwide program is needed to stop the spread of the disease.

581. Mann, Jonathan M. et al. "The International Epidemiology of AIDS." Scientific American, v. 259, October 1988, pp. 82-89.

At least five million people worldwide are currently infected by the AIDS virus. Over one million new cases of the disease will be reported in the next five years. The geographic distribution of the disease is presented.

582. McTigue, James F. "The United States and the International Control of AIDS." <u>Annals of the American Academy of Political and Social Science</u>, v. 500, November 1988, pp. 91-104.

AIDS presents different epidemiological problems in different parts of the world. The economic and social consequences of AIDS are also having a profound impact on many nations. An international effort is required to stop the spread of the disease. The United States must take a leadership role in AIDS research, information sharing, and education.

583. "Namibia Fears AIDS Epidemic From Peace Troops and Returning Refugees." <u>New Scientist</u>, v. 120, December 17, 1988, p. 8.

The peace settlement in Namibia may result in the introduction of an AIDS epidemic in that nation. The government would like to screen all returning refugees and the United Nations peacekeeping forces in order to prevent infected individuals from entering the country.

584. "New Model Predicts Future HIV in Africa." <u>New Scientist</u>, v. 119, September 22, 1988, p. 28.

A new model of the spread of AIDS indicates that there may be ten times as many cases of AIDS in Africa as have previously been reported. This model agrees well with the current number of American and European cases.

585. "Passage of Recommendations Allows CMA to Release Policy Statement on AIDS." <u>Canadian Medical Association Journal</u>, v. 139, September 15, 1988, pp. 545-549.

The Canadian Medical Association had a spirited debate about AIDS at its annual conference. It passed a recommendation that AIDS testing be carried out with informed consent whenever possible. Six other AIDS statements and policies were also approved.

586. Patrushev, Pyotr. "AIDS Tests Soviet Tolerance." <u>World Press Review</u>, v. 35, December 1988, p. 54.

AIDS is having significant social and psychological repercussions in the Soviet Union. Members of high risk groups are experiencing discrimination. Education is needed to inform the public about the facts of the disease.

587. "Poles Told to Bring Their Own Syringes." <u>New Scientist</u>, v. 119, July 7, 1988, p. 32.

Lack of funding is inhibiting the Polish fight against AIDS. The government cannot afford to pay for testing to ensure the safety of the blood supply. Health officials feel that the biggest danger for the spread of the virus is through prostitution.

588. Romano, Nino et al. "Main Routes of Transmission of Human Immunodeficiency Virus (HIV) Infection in a Family Setting in Palermo, Italy." <u>American Journal of Epidemiology</u>, v. 128, August 1988, pp. 254-260.
     In a survey of personal contacts of drug abusers with AIDS, none of the nonsexual contacts tested positive. Six of 36 sexual partners and four children were infected. There is a high rate of vertical transmission from mother to child, an intermediate rate among sexual partners, and no risk to casual contacts.

589. Ross, Michael W. "Distribution of Knowledge of AIDS: A National Study." <u>Social Sciences and Medicine</u>, v. 27, 1988, pp. 1295-1298.
     Over 2,600 Australians were surveyed to determine their knowledge level about AIDS. Individuals with lower knowledge levels had a greater fear of homosexuals, were more unrealistic about AIDS, and placed more blame on the victims.

590. **Sabatier, Renee and Judith Mariasy. "AIDS in Africa."** <u>**Christianity and Crisis**</u>, **v. 48, July 4, 1988, pp. 232-235.**
     AIDS has become epidemic in some parts of Africa, reaching an incidence rate similar to that in the United States. However, African economies often cannot afford to care for AIDS patients because the costs of treatment are so high. Education programs must be established to stop the spread of the disease.

591. Seftel, David. "AIDS and Apartheid: Double Trouble." <u>Africa Report</u>, v. 33, November/December 1988, pp. 17-22.
     The nation of South Africa provides unequal medical services for Blacks and Whites. Blacks receive poorer health care, which can be fatal when dealing with AIDS. The use of migrant workers and the lack of screening of blood for Blacks has helped to spread the disease in this population.

592. Seidel, Gill. "A Very Special Relationship." <u>New Statesman and Society</u>, v. 1, October 7, 1988, pp. 21-22.
     A new AIDS education and counselling program has been established in Uganda. This program emphasizes the encouragement of a positive attitude towards AIDS patients instead of avoidance.

593. Sepulveda, Jaime. "AIDS in Mexico." <u>World Health</u>, July 1988, pp. 18-19.
     The initial cases of AIDS in Mexico all involved individuals who had some contact with persons in the United States. However, the disease has now spread throughout the nation and over 1,000 cases have been reported. Over 90% of the victims are homosexual or bisexual men. Educational programs have been established to prevent the further spread of the disease.

594. "Sex Change in Uganda." Economist, v. 308, August 13, 1988, p. 38.

   Uganda is one of nations that has been hit the hardest by the AIDS epidemic. An AIDS education program has successfully reduced the spread of the disease in this nation.

595. Stiles, B. J. "Talking AIDS in Stockholm." Christianity and Crisis, v. 48, August 1, 1988, pp. 63-64.

   Sweden has reported fewer than 200 cases of AIDS, but that nation is working hard to stop the spread of the virus. The Fourth International Conference on AIDS was recently held in Sweden to discuss scientific advances in the battle against the disease.

596. Tinker, Jon. "AIDS in the Developing Countries." Issues in Science and Technology, v. 4, Winter 1988, pp. 43-48.

   AIDS has become a worldwide epidemic that is most devastating to Third World nations. Those countries not only suffer the medical problems of AIDS, but they also do not have the economic base to pay for the therapies and preventions used in some of the more developed nations.

597. "UNESCO's Action on AIDS." Impact of Science on Society, no. 150, 1988, pp. 169-170.

   UNESCO has adopted a policy authorizing the organization to support national and regional AIDS programs. UNESCO will work with schools to establish effective AIDS education programs.

598. United States. Congress. House. Select Committee on Hunger. AIDS and the Third World: The Impact on Development. Washington, D.C.: Government Printing Office, 1988. 115p. Superintendent of Documents number Y4.H89:100-29.

   The complete text of a Senate hearing on the effects of AIDS on the Third World, with particular emphasis on Africa. The United States must assist international organizations in helping to stop the spread of AIDS in other nations whose resources are inadequate to fight the disease.

599. Wahren, Carl. "Can AIDS Be Contained?" OECD Observer, no. 154, October/November 1988, pp. 22-27.

   As of July 1988, over 100,000 cases of AIDS have been reported worldwide. The virus is spread through sexual contact and intravenous drug abuse. There is currently no vaccine or cure. Over 100 nations have initiated AIDS control programs.

600. Walters, David. "Managing the AIDS Epidemic: The Canadian Report Card." Canadian Journal of Public Health, v. 79, September/October 1988, pp. 293-295.

   While the Canadian health system has responded well to the AIDS epidemic, more effort is needed in monitoring the incidence of the disease. In many areas related to AIDS, Canada falls in the shadow of the United States, which has an overwhelmingly greater number of cases.

601. Watson, Catharine. "An Open Approach to AIDS." Africa Report, v. 33, November/December 1988, pp. 32-34.

Uganda has one of the world's worst AIDS epidemics, but it has also been one of the most open African nations about this problem. A strong AIDS education program has helped to dramatically slow the rate of infection.

602. Widy-Wirski, Roslaw et al. "Evaluation of the WHO Clinical Case Definition for AIDS in Uganda." JAMA: Journal of the American Medical Association, v. 260, December 9, 1988, pp. 3286-3289.

In order to test the World Health Organization case definition for AIDS in Third World nations, 1,328 patients were tested in fifteen hospitals in Uganda. Over 40% of the patients tested positive using the ELISA blood test. With the exception of the need for the addition of amenorrhea to the case definition for female victims, the existing case definition is accurate.

603. Wilson-Smith, Anthony. "AIDS in Russia." Maclean's, v. 101, December 12, 1988, pp. 58-59.

A Soviet prostitute was the first person to die of AIDS in that nation. Although authorities blame foreigners for introducing the virus into the country, they now admit that AIDS has become a serious problem.

604. Wood, William B. "AIDS North and South: Diffusion Patterns of a Global Epidemic and a Research Agenda for Geographers." Professional Geographer, v. 40, August 1988, pp. 266-279.

The groups at risk for AIDS and the spatial patterns of its distribution vary considerably from one region to another. The distribution of AIDS in North America and Europe is very different from that in Africa and the Caribbean. Geographers will be needed to analyze the global distribution and spread of the disease.

The Future of the AIDS Epidemic

605. Connor, Steve. "Poor Data Hamper Predictions on AIDS." New Scientist, v. 120, December 10, 1988, p. 14.

Between 20,000 and 50,000 persons were infected by the AIDS virus by the end of 1987. Three models of the future of the AIDS crisis give three different projections, but each is hampered by uncertainty about the current number of cases.

606. Francis, Donald P. "Prospects for the Future." Death Studies, v. 12, 1988, pp. 597-607.

No cure for AIDS will be found within the next five years, although some treatments to reduce suffering will be discovered. Most of the cases in the United States and Europe will continue to be among members of high-risk groups. Education programs will help slow the spread of the disease to other groups.

607. Fumento, Michael. "The AIDS Numbers Racket: Chapter 37." National Review, v. 40, October 14, 1988, pp. 45+.

A new report states that as many as 1.9 million Americans may have become infected by the AIDS virus through the end of 1987. This is twice the estimates made by the Centers for Disease Control. The statistical methods behind this study are flawed and were used only to generate sensational reports for the media.

608. Newmark, Peter. "AIDS Predictions Until 1992." Nature, v. 336, December 8, 1988, p. 508.

At least 10,000 new cases of AIDS have been predicted to appear in Great Britain by 1992. Under-reporting of the current state of the disease may account for as many as 40% additional cases.

Animal Models for AIDS and AIDS in Animals

609. "Animal Models for HIV Infection and AIDS: Memorandum From a WHO Meeting." _Bulletin of the World Health Organization_, v. 66, 1988, pp. 561-574.

Three major animal models are currently available for the study of AIDS: the simian immunodeficiency virus, non-primate lentiviruses, and HIV infection of non-human primates. These animal models are critical for the development of vaccines and drug therapies for AIDS.

610. Ezzell, Carol. "Laboratory Accident Kills AIDS Mice." _Nature_, v. 336, December 15, 1988, p. 613.

The first study of AIDS in mice ended when the mice died in a laboratory accident. The ventilation was turned off in the laboratory and the mice died from accidental overheating.

611. "Gabon Isolates Chimp Virus." _New Scientist_, v. 119, September 22, 1988, p. 29.

African researchers have isolated a virus from chimpanzees that is similar to the human AIDS virus. There is no evidence that the people who live in the same geographic regions as the chimpanzees can also become infected.

612. Hendricks, Melissa. "Human Immune System Implanted in Mice." _Science News_, v. 134, September 24, 1988, p. 198.

Two research groups have successfully genetically engineered the human immune system into mice. This may provide an animal model for the study of AIDS and other immune system disorders.

613. Kingman, Sharon. "Japanese Cats Risk AIDS From Nights Out." _New Scientist_, v. 119, July 7, 1988, p. 34.

Of 3,000 cats tested for the feline immunodeficiency virus in Tokyo, approximately 30% tested positive. This virus is spread through scratching or biting and is becoming epidemic among cats in this city.

614. Langone, John. "Of Mice As Stand-Ins for Men." _Time_, v. 132, September 26, 1988, p. 70.

Two researchers have successfully transplanted parts of the human immune system into mice. These mice can now be used to study human diseases such as AIDS. The mice can also be used as testing grounds for new drugs and treatments.

615. Marx, Jean L. "AIDS Mice Die in NIH Accident." _Science_, v. 242, December 16, 1988, p. 1502.

A laboratory accident has killed all but three of 130 mice used in an AIDS research program. The mice died when the electricity to the building was shut off for maintenance work.

616. Marx, Jean L.   "Progress Reported on Mouse Models for AIDS."   _Science_, v. 242, December 23, 1988, p. 1638.
     The lack of an animal model has hindered some AIDS research.   Three groups of researchers have developed mice that carry the AIDS virus.   These mice may enable researchers to conduct some AIDS experiments in animals.

617. "The Mouse's Tale."   _Economist_, v. 308, July 16, 1988, p. 82.
     Scientists have recently been able to breed mice who carry the genes of the AIDS virus.   These mice develop the symptoms of AIDS even though the virus does not kill their cells.

618. "Of Mice and Medicine Men."   _Newsweek_, v. 112, September 26, 1988, p. 70.
     Two researchers have announced that they have successfully engineered a virus that produces AIDS in mice. This may create an animal model for the study of AIDS.

619. "Of Mice and Men."   _U.S. News and World Report_, v. 105, September 26, 1988, p. 11.
     Two research teams have recently been able to introduce human immune system components into mice.   This opens the door for the use of mice in the fight against AIDS.

620. Revkin, Andrew C.   "The Search for an Animal Model." _Discover_, v. 9, November 1988, pp. 6-7.
     Medical researchers have not yet been able to find an effective animal model for AIDS.   Chimpanzees can become infected by the human AIDS virus, but they don't get the disease.   Two research groups have genetically engineered a virus that can be used to study AIDS in mice and rabbits.

621. Weiss, Rick.   "First Mutant Mice Infected With AIDS." _Science News_, v. 134, December 24, 1988, p. 404.
     Researchers have been successful in introducing AIDS into mice who have been genetically engineered to model the human immune system.   This provides the first animal model for AIDS.

622. Weiss, Robin A.   "Novel HIV Systems."   _Nature_, v. 335, October 13, 1988, p. 591.
     Scientists have long sought animal models for AIDS.   Some attempts to modify the virus to infect rabbits and mice are described.

Peter Duesberg and the Non-Viral Theory of AIDS

623. Blattner, W., Robert C. Gallo, and H. M. Temin. "HIV Causes AIDS." <u>Science</u>, v. 241, July 29, 1988, p. 515.

The AIDS virus is suspected of causing the disease because the virus has been linked to all groups with the disease. The introduction of the virus into a population is essential for the introduction of the disease. The virus has also been directly linked with transfusion-associated AIDS.

624. Duesberg, Peter. "HIV Is Not the Cause of AIDS." <u>Science</u>, v. 241, July 29, 1988, p. 514.

The AIDS virus does not cause AIDS because it fails several standard medical postulates. The virus cannot be isolated from all cases, it does not trigger the disease in all infected persons, it is not biochemically active in the disease, and there is an extremely long time period between initial infection and the onset of the disease.

Author Index

References are to entry numbers and not to page numbers.

Subject Index

Prepared by Linda Webster

Italicized numbers are page numbers; all other numbers are entry numbers.